T0209437

ADDICTION
the Dark Night of the Soul

NAD+
the Light of Hope

Paula Norris Mestayer

BALBOA.
PRESS
A DIVISION OF HAY HOUSE

Copyright © 2018 Paula Norris Mestayer.

All rights reserved. No part of this book may be used or reproduced by
any means, graphic, electronic, or mechanical, including photocopying,
recording, taping or by any information storage retrieval system
without the written permission of the author except in the case of
brief quotations embodied in critical articles and reviews.

Balboa Press books may be ordered through booksellers or by contacting:

Balboa Press
A Division of Hay House
1663 Liberty Drive
Bloomington, IN 47403
www.balboapress.com
1 (877) 407-4847

Because of the dynamic nature of the Internet, any web addresses or
links contained in this book may have changed since publication and
may no longer be valid. The views expressed in this work are solely those
of the author and do not necessarily reflect the views of the publisher,
and the publisher hereby disclaims any responsibility for them.

The author of this book does not dispense medical advice or prescribe the use
of any technique as a form of treatment for physical, emotional, or medical
problems without the advice of a physician, either directly or indirectly. The
intent of the author is only to offer information of a general nature to help
you in your quest for emotional and spiritual well-being. In the event you use
any of the information in this book for yourself, which is your constitutional
right, the author and the publisher assume no responsibility for your actions.

Any people depicted in stock imagery provided by Getty Images are
models, and such images are being used for illustrative purposes only.
Certain stock imagery © Getty Images.

Print information available on the last page.

ISBN: 978-1-9822-1813-3 (sc)
ISBN: 978-1-9822-1815-7 (hc)
ISBN: 978-1-9822-1814-0 (e)

Library of Congress Control Number: 2018914885

Balboa Press rev. date: 01/15/2019

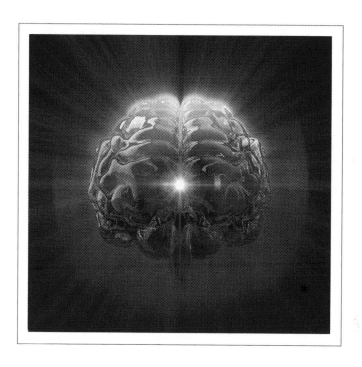

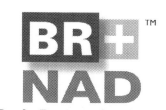

Brain Restoration Plus
Nicotinamide Adenine Dinucleotide

The future of brain health

Dedicated to Love
from my family and friends
especially the love manifested through
the lives of my father and mother,
Col. Willard and Ruth Norris

"Love adds a precious seeing to the eye."
—William Shakespeare

Contents

Foreword

Elizabeth A. Stuller, MD

In my work as a Board-Certified Adult and Addiction Psychiatrist, I have had the unique opportunity to collaborate with Paula Norris Mestayer on our mutual patients, both on a personal and professional level. I am pleased to write the forward to this book in part because the contents of the book have helped me in my clinical practice.

Paula Norris Mestayer is a "Woman of Substance" by Southern terms, whose very presence commands an admirable respect of doctors and patients alike. What has been most striking to me as a keen observer of human behavior is Paula's incredible talent in counseling the very complex psychiatric and addicted patient. She is skillful and tactical in getting to the root cause of psychological pathology in an efficient yet compassionate way, leaving the patient feeling quite hopeful and nicely disarmed. In the treatment of our complex dual diagnosis patients with comorbid personality disorders, Paula is extremely professional in maintaining the delicate line of professional boundaries while remaining helpful and therapeutic. I would say in my professional career, without any doubt, that Paula is by far the most skillful therapist I have had the pleasure of observing. She remains open and willing to take on the patient whom many a psychiatrist might have abandoned at their own wits' end.

Paula has many feathers in her cap, including her proficiency as a mother, writer, business woman, researcher, and entrepreneur. I often say that Paula has the skill set to run small countries in her spare time. Despite her repertoire of abilities, she remains a humble human servant whose kind smile and words act as a healing balm for many souls.

It is therefore without reservation that I highly recommend Paula's first book, *Addiction: The Dark Night of the Soul; NAD+: The Light of Hope.* It is the treatise of her personal and professional journey with Nicotinamide Adenine Dinucleotide (NAD+). She and her husband, Dr. Richard Mestayer, III, hold the distinction of having administered Intravenous (IV) NAD+ treatment longer than anyone else in the United States. Paula Norris Mestayer is the founder of Springfield Wellness Center and the most experienced psychotherapist and counselor in the use of IV NAD+. Without a doubt, Paula will always remain an eager, ready learner with childlike enthusiasm and robust energy in her pursuit of continued excellence in her field and goal of advancing NAD+ in addiction and mental health treatment.

Preface

This is a book about addiction and brain restoration. It is about an epidemic sweeping our country, taking millions of Americans through a personal and collective "dark night of the soul."

I wouldn't be writing this book if that was the only focus. Instead, it's to share with you what I've learned from personal experience and nearly 40 years of clinical practice: that there is a way out of our addiction nightmare as well as the nightmare of the debilitating consequences of cognitive decline associated with aging, injuries suffered from combat, accidents, and concussions suffered from rough contact sports. It takes the form of a natural, non-narcotic substance that can restore the brain. This ubiquitous little coenzyme of niacin—called coenzyme 1 of Vitamin B3—can break the rehab/relapse cycle of addition and give people their lives back, as well as giving HOPE to those with a multiplicity of other neurological concerns. The process doesn't involve an agonizing withdrawal; nor does it leave the patient with intolerable cravings. In fact, most people hear about it and say, "It sounds too good to be true." Then they experience it, or witness it, and learn what I know:

It is true!

And here is why. That ubiquitous little coenzyme is an "essential bio-nutrient" for cellular health. It is as essential to our health as oxygen.

In the pages of this book I'm going to share with you what

I've seen; the clinical results I've witnessed; and what I know of the ongoing research that is explaining why and how our intravenous BR+NAD™ treatment works. When you finish reading, I hope you'll become an ambassador for a conversation that can change the course of neurodegenerative diseases and addiction treatment in our country. There's no reason to prolong our national addiction nightmare. There's no reason to substitute one narcotic for another and call it therapy. Instead, it's time to recognize that addiction is a brain disease and when you give the brain what it needs to recover, it does. No more dependence; no more cravings; no more pain. The dark night of the soul is over. As the saying goes,

"The darkest hour is just before dawn."

It's morning again. The sun is rising. It is a new day!

Acknowledgements

(alphabetical order)

Michelle Aycock
Miranda Baham
Debra Neill Baker
Pat Becker
James Bennett
Kim & Charles Bienvenu
Jade Berg, PhD
Hedy Boelte
Nady Braidy, PhD
Dan Brown, PhD
Jo Ann Brumfield
Vera Bryant
Mr. and Mrs. Van Ness Butler
Van Butler
Sam, Carl, Stephen Camp
Ron Campton
Louis Cataldie MD
Gurumayi Chidvilasananda
Lucy Colclough
Richard Colon
Doug Cook, MD
Lourdes Corbala

David Cuccia, MD
André de la Barre
Karla and Matt Diehl
Jane Downe
Dave and Brenda Dooley
Melissa Dufrene
Jason Faciane
Charles Kronlage, Esq.
Lara Galloway
Susan Broom-Gibson, PhD
Leslee Goodman
Billy Gorman
Cheryl Grace
Keith Graham
Ross Grant, PhD
Norris and Patsy Gremillion
Matt Hardy
Dean Hickman, MD
Melody Hite
William Hitt
Paula Hotard
John La Martina, MD
Lidonna Lancaster, MD
David Lefer, PhD
Arlene Magee
John Melhorne
Rachael Murphy, MD
Richard F. Mestayer, III, MD
Theresa Norris
Tyson Olds, MD
Stan Owen, MD
Beverly & Pam Oxenrider
Jeanne Petri
Tiffany Noel Phillips

Garland Robinette
Ann Rogers
Darren Scoggins
Linni Silberman
Karen Simone
Tom Steinitz
Judy Storch
Elizabeth Stuller, MD
Sherry Summers
James Watson, MD
Tom Ubl
Sue Vacarro
Keith Vicknair
Carrie Wibright
Ray Wilkes

Staff at Archway Apothecary
Staff at Equipoise Wellness
Staff at the William Hitt Center
Staff at Springfield Wellness Center (past and present)

All the patients who taught me so much and whose
souls are connected to mine in perpetuity

CHAPTER ONE

Southern Dumb Belle

As I know from personal experience, the dark night of the soul is the painful and terrifying dissolution of all that one believes in, lives by, lives for, considers one's purpose, and defines oneself as. It is a sense of meaninglessness so vast it feels like floating in a dark space without gravity to indicate up or down. ALONE! No beginning and no end, just suspended in the word "why," hoping for an answer, which doesn't come until at last it is over and you are no longer floating. It is an existential crisis of the ultimate betrayal. At least that is how I defined mine. Where was the God I believed in? Why would He allow me to feel this terror when I had kept my covenant? Was this a punishment for sins I didn't even know I'd committed? Why me? I'd always strived to be "good." Does God really exist after all? If He doesn't, what can I hold on to? Nothingness? Is this really all there is? Are all my concepts of self and other and meaning and faith just products of my conditioning?

The dark night of the soul often follows some tragic event for which there is no satisfactory explanation. So far, my life has given me two dark nights. The first, which I will share now, began in 1975. The second, which I will hold for another time, began in 1992. The first was the death of my father and the death of my marriage within a few months of each other. While I was reeling from the narcissistic wound of my husband leaving me for another woman, my father, my hero, died suddenly, leaving my mother and me to grieve separately but together in our own personal darkness. We each eventually found our way out, but not without significant personal effort. Now that the two men I loved and admired most were no longer in my life, I began my odyssey to redefine myself by searching for the answer to the question, "Why?"

The length of time a dark night lasts varies from person to person, as does the number of dark-night episodes one might have. My work with those who suffer from the scourge of addiction reveals that dark nights can last for years, or even for a lifetime.

St. John of the Cross believed that the dark night of the soul was God's way of perfecting us. A Spanish poet and mystic born in 1542 and canonized in 1726, St. John of the Cross was a Carmelite priest who worked with St. Teresa of Avila to reform the Order. He suffered greatly at the hands of his brother Carmelites when they imprisoned and tortured him for his attempts at reformation. Nine months later he escaped from prison, where he wrote his famous poem, *Dark Night of the Soul*, detailing the excruciating despair of his ego-death when he nearly lost his faith.

"Being perfected through suffering" was not the kind of belief I held before going through my own dark night, but I can confess now that these anguished periods were the best things that ever happened to me. It is during these times that we are the most egoless. Our pain is so deep that we barely exist, wandering around in disbelief trying to redefine who we are. From that, wisdom is born.

Several memorable events took place during my time of searching. One, in particular, is the reason I am even writing this book about NAD+ and why I risked so much to bring it back to the United States.

I began to come out of this dark night by returning to school for a second graduate degree, this time in psychotherapy. I had neatly identified this as the perfect way to find the answers I was searching for, without having to expose my vulnerabilities to a therapist. I'd study the psyche *in general*, rather than having to reveal mine or so I thought.

I was accepted to a unique program through Tulane University in which I did most of my coursework on campus, but the specialty courses I wanted to take were offered in the summer at Connecticut College and Duke University. These were followed by a six-month internship in New York at the Manhattan Children's Psychiatric Hospital.

My excitement at being accepted overshadowed my responsibilities at the time. I was in the middle of renovating my first house and had two weeks to shut down the renovation, ship my three dogs to my mother, and pack for a summer in New London, Connecticut. Those two weeks sped by, and before I knew it, I was off the plane and in a taxi on my way to Connecticut College. Wow, what a whirlwind.

The taxi driver, interestingly, was going through a divorce, too, so I was very capable of empathizing and "sharing his pain," as my own divorce was less than a year old.

I got out of the taxi and carried my luggage to the dorm, when it hit me. Out of nowhere came a surge of anxiety that stopped me in my tracks. My joy and excitement had successfully hidden my fear of academia. Here I was in a strange town, alone, about to face a summer of learning in an Ivy League environment, when all I knew were LSU and Tulane—both schools in the Deep South. My fear of being "found out," that I might not be smart enough to compete academically, came crashing down on me. I was certain I would be out of place and looked upon negatively because of the unfair perceptions of the South that are held by some in the East. In fact, a verse from a Randy Newman song about LSU, "where they go in dumb and come out dumb, too," kept skipping like a scratched record in my mind. I had always felt insecure academically, but I hid it very well—or so I thought. Even though the "smart kids" always wanted to play or hang out with me and my teachers gave me good grades, I thought I had merely fooled them all into thinking I was smart.

So here I was standing at the front desk of the dorm, receiving my key and room number while thoughts of running home and getting my money back swirled in my head. I walked timidly down the long hall, scanning each door for my number, and taking deep breaths as I inserted the key into the door that was mine. I opened the door, walked in, dropped my luggage, and leaned back against the door as it closed. I was terrified. How was I going to be able to get through this semester? I started crying. I was on my own; utterly alone. My fear and sadness were indistinguishable; both emotions were swirling so fast they became one. I just cried, leaning against the door, which I can feel again merely by writing this.

What happened next is hard to believe, but it is the unadulterated truth.

I told myself to straighten up, get a grip, and then I prayed something like, "Please, God, oh please, please let me know I am doing the right thing. Please, I know it is silly, but give me a sign that I am where I am supposed to be and doing what I am supposed to do." I paused for a moment, not really expecting a response, before deciding that I would open the beautiful draperies covering the large window and check out the view. I crossed the room, drew back the draperies, and saw a magnificent blue spruce perfectly framed by the window. My thought was a question: Is this my sign? It didn't feel like a sign, so I shrugged it off and, just as I began to walk away, looked down and saw a single word carved into the window frame.

"PAULA," my name, in all capital letters. Yes, I was meant to be here.

So, what does a stunned young woman from the South do when something like this happens? She starts laughing gratefully, accepting the answered prayer as a gift and a sign that she is on the right path. That path has led me to help many others experiencing their dark nights of the soul, wrestling with the plague of addiction, depression, anxiety or bereavement. Having "walked through the Valley of the Shadow of Death" with so many of them, I can tell you for certain there is light on the other side.

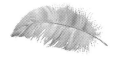

"There is no dishonor in losing the race. There is only dishonor in not racing because you are afraid to lose."
—Garth Stein

CHAPTER TWO

Wrestling with Addiction: Our Collective Dark Night

The United States is in the grip of a lethal epidemic. It's an outbreak that affects virtually every American family and that claims more lives each year than traffic accidents, homicides, and suicides combined. It often takes adults in the prime of their lives, or even younger, and turns them into desperate skeletons, cruel caricatures of their former selves. Before it kills them, it typically destroys them in other ways: stripping them of dignity and self-respect; taking their hopes, their jobs, their families, their friends. It often results in the loss of their houses, their cars, their savings, if they have any. If their disease causes them to run afoul of law enforcement, rather than the medical establishment, it also takes their freedom. Perhaps worst of all, it takes their future. With few effective treatment options—and no cures—its victims believe they are locked in a hopeless battle with this disease for the rest of their lives.

The epidemic, of course, is addiction, and experts say there is virtually no family in America that isn't dealing with it—or the tragic aftermath of it, because all too often family members find out about this illness when it has killed someone they love.

According to the National Survey on Drug Use and Health (NSDUH), 21.5 million American adults (aged 12 and older) battled a substance use disorder in 2014.[1] The NSDUH is the primary source for statistical information on illicit drug use, alcohol use, substance use disorders (SUDs), mental health issues, and co-occurring SUDs and mental health issues for the civilian, noninstitutionalized population of the United States. Its results are, therefore, probably low, as they exclude members of the military, as well as people in hospitals, rehab facilities, prisons, and other institutions.

Adults with "alcohol use disorder" (AUD) topped the charts at 17.0 million civilians. Adolescents 12-17 with AUD added another 679,000.[2] The addiction that is getting all the media attention, however, is to prescription opiates, which claimed an astonishing 2.1 million adults in 2012, while an additional 467,000 Americans were addicted to the street opiate, heroin.[3] Third on the list—and in some ways far more frightening because of the speed at which it kills—was the number of "regular" methamphetamine users: 1.5 million. Another frightening figure: 1.1 million kids aged 12-17 had used inhalants at least once in the past 12 months, and a whopping 59% of them had at least one friend who "was using an inhalant on a regular basis."[4]

Although the study didn't include estimates for the number of adults abusing benzodiazepines (central nervous system depressants like Valium and Xanax), researchers can tell us that more than 33,000 Americans were hospitalized for

---

[1] Behavioral Health Trends in the United States: Results from the 2014 National Survey on Drug Use and Health, Substance Abuse and Mental Health Services Administration, Department of Health and Human Services, September 2015.

[2] https://www.niaaa.nih.gov/alcohol-health/overview-alcohol-consumption/alcohol-facts-and-statistics

[3] Substance Abuse and Mental Health Services Administration, Results from the 2012 National Survey on Drug Use and Health: Summary of National Findings, NSDUH Series H-46, HHS Publication No. (SMA) 13-4795. Rockville, MD: Substance Abuse and Mental Health Services Administration, 2013

[4] http://healthresearchfunding.org/24-shocking-inhalant-abuse-statistics/

benzodiazepine overdose in 2012 and that more than *50 million* prescriptions for these sedatives are written in the U.S. each year.[5]

Compounding addiction's tragic effects are that it's an illness for which people are ashamed to seek treatment. A 2015 study by Columbia University found that "Only one in 10 people with addiction to alcohol and/or drugs report receiving any treatment at all. Compare this to the fact that about 70 percent of people with hypertension or diabetes do receive treatment. Can you imagine accepting that degree of neglect if that were the case for heart or lung disease, cancer, asthma, diabetes, tuberculosis, stroke and other diseases of the brain?"[6]

There are various reasons for individuals' reluctance to seek medical care, most related in some way to the issue of shame: shame to admit they're addicted and need help; fear they won't be able to beat the addiction, thereby increasing their feelings of failure and inadequacy. They're also fearful of the cost of treatment and worried that their health insurance won't cover it—because it's a character defect, a lifestyle choice, not an illness. Then, too, in the case of opiates and benzodiazepines, it was the medical establishment that got them addicted in the first place—and, as they grew increasingly tolerant, and then addicted, cut them off. Finally, addicts have little hope that treatment will work. They've heard too many stories of treatment being just another revolving door: in a matter of months, the patients relapse; addiction wins again.

Why is America facing this epidemic? Why are millions of people seeking the relief of addictive narcotics to function in our world?

---

[5] https://www.addictioncenter.com/benzodiazepines/
https://www.addictionhope.com/benzodiazepine/
https://www.drugabuse.gov/sites/default/files/rrprescription.pdf
[6] http://www.usnews.com/opinion/blogs/policy-dose/2015/06/01/
america-is-neglecting-its-addiction-problem

Pain is a significant factor. According to a recent Institute of Medicine report, some 100 million Americans live with chronic pain[7] including low back pain (28.1% of chronic pain sufferers), severe headache or migraine (16.1%), neck pain (15.1%), knee pain (19.5%), shoulder pain (9.0%), finger pain (7.6%), and hip pain (7.1%). Because everything in the body is connected, most pain sufferers experience pain at multiple sites: low back pain leads to pain in the hips and legs; neck pain leads to headaches or migraines, etc. (ibid) Other common causes of chronic pain include cancer, arthritis, and neurogenic pain, which is pain resulting from damage to the peripheral nerves or to the central nervous system itself. This type of pain alone is at epidemic proportions according to Tina Tockarshewsky, of the Neuropathy Association, who said "More than 6 million Americans have unrelenting nerve pain. Now it will increase tremendously because of the epidemic of diabetes." (ibid)

Large as these numbers are, they continue to understate the level of pain we are collectively experiencing as a people. They don't include pain in children, for example, or pain-related conditions such as lupus, sickle-cell disease, ankylosing spondylitis, and others. Also, both the NHIS and the NHANES studies "use samples of civilian, noninstitutionalized populations. They do not include people with chronic pain who are in the military or live in corrections facilities, nursing homes, or other chronic care facilities." (ibid)

---

[7] National Academies Press: Relieving Pain in America: A Blueprint for Transforming Prevention, Care, Education, and Research (2011) https://www.nap.edu/read/13172/chapter/4#61 (*The major sources of U.S. population health data including information on pain are two large, ongoing surveys conducted by the National Center for Health Statistics (NCHS), an agency within CDC. The first is the National Health Interview Survey (NHIS), an ongoing, cross-sectional household interview survey of approximately 35,000 U.S. households collectively containing about 87,500 persons. It is large enough to enable analysis of health information for many demographic and socioeconomic groups. The second is the National Health and Nutrition Examination Survey (NHANES), which collects data through in-person interviews and physical examinations of a representative sample of about 5,000 Americans annually.*)

As a healthcare provider treating people with addiction, acute and chronic pain, as well as post-traumatic stress, I can confirm that our veterans are returning from combat overseas with very high levels of pain—physical, psychic, and emotional. If millions of *civilians* are experiencing chronic pain, undoubtedly a high percentage of members of our military is also suffering—in VA hospitals and while still on active duty.

And the incidence of chronic pain is likely only to get worse. First, we're getting older, which means that more Americans will experience diseases associated with chronic pain—diabetes, cardiovascular disorders, arthritis, and cancer, among others. (ibid, Cherry et al., 2010)

Second, we're getting fatter, and obesity leads to chronic conditions with painful symptoms, such as diabetes-associated neuropathy, and orthopedic problems, including cartilage degradation. (ibid, Richettel et al., 2011) As a result, more Americans will have joint replacement surgeries and at younger ages. (ibid, Harms et al., 2007; Changulani et al., 2008) These surgeries themselves can sometimes cause persistent pain that interferes with a full recovery and a resumed quality of life. Obesity also is associated with higher rates of other types of pain, notably migraine. (ibid, Peterlin et al., 2009)

Third, as the Committee on Advancing Pain Research, Care, and Education points out, progress in saving the lives of people with catastrophic injuries related to work, sports, car accidents, or military combat who would have died in decades past, creates growing numbers of relatively young people at high risk of lifelong chronic pain. Similarly, modern medicine can help many people with serious illnesses survive longer, but the cost of survival may be debilitating pain. Cancer chemotherapy, for example, can save a life but result in neuropathic pain.

Fourth, all surgical patients are at risk of both acute and chronic pain as a result of their surgery. Currently, about 60% of surgical procedures in the U.S. are performed on an outpatient basis, where persistent problems with adequate pain control after ambulatory surgery are well documented. The most significant risk of undermanaged acute postsurgical pain is that it may develop into chronic pain. (ibid, Rawal, 2007; Schug and Chong, 2009)

Back pain is the leading cause of disability in Americans under 45 years old. More than 26 million Americans between the ages of 20-64 experience frequent back pain.[8]

A study of chronic low back pain conducted in North Carolina found "an alarming increase in the prevalence of chronic [low back pain] from 1992 to 2006 … across all population subgroups." The prevalence for the total population studied more than doubled over the period, from about 4% to more than 10%, and for women (all ages) and men aged 45-54, prevalence nearly tripled.[9] Although these data are from a single state, a similar growth pattern has been seen in national data for users of the Department of Veterans Affairs health system, which show an annualized increase in the prevalence of low back pain of about 5% per year, more substantial than increases in three other conditions studied (depression, diabetes, and hypertension).[10]

Aside from those injured in war or accidents, our sedentary lifestyle—compounded by obesity—may explain why so many Americans are now experiencing intractable back pain. The human body was designed to move, not sit still. Dr. James Levine, director of the Mayo Clinic-Arizona State University's Obesity Solutions Initiative, has been studying the adverse

---

[8] National Centers for Health Statistics, Chartbook on Trends in the Health of Americans 2006, Special Feature: Pain

[9] Janet K. Freburger, PT, PhD; George M. Holmes, PhD; Robert P. Agans, PhD; et al, The rising prevalence of chronic low back pain, *Arch Intern Med.* 2009;169(3):251-258. doi:10.1001/archinternmed.2008.543

[10] Patricia Sinnott, PT, PhD, MPH; Todd H. Wagner, PhD, Low Back Pain in VA Users, *Arch Intern Med.* 2009;169(14):1336-1340. doi:10.1001/archinternmed.2009.201

effects of our increasingly sedentary lifestyles for years and has summed up his findings in two sentences.

"Sitting is more dangerous than smoking, kills more people than HIV, and is more treacherous than parachuting. We are sitting ourselves to death."[11]

While research shows that prolonged sitting contributes to life-shortening diseases like cancer, depression, heart disease, and Type 2 diabetes, it also causes musculature changes that, over time, can be debilitating. Not surprisingly, many of these involve the neck and low back.

There are other questions we might ask ourselves to achieve greater insight into why so many of us need to anesthetize ourselves. Why, for example, do 40 million of us—18 percent of the adult population—experience anxiety disorder in any 12-month period?[12] We're not talking about occasional anxiety—which is an appropriate response to certain life situations—but anxiety *disorders*, which include post-traumatic stress, obsessive-compulsive disorder, panic disorder, social anxiety disorder, and others. Another question we might ask ourselves is "Why do physicians prescribe a drug to ease the feelings of anxiety, rather than attempt to understand what is making us feel this way?"

I believe we are collectively experiencing a dark night of the soul. We're working harder and harder at a life that does not satisfy. And as any addict can tell you, you can never get enough of that which does not satisfy.

I've been through my own dark nights of the soul and, excruciating as they are, they've taught me a lot. In fact, they were a significant reason I chose to be a psychotherapist. Few people want to experience their agonizing dark nights. We're a "quick fix" nation. If something is troubling us, our default response

---

[11] http://www.latimes.com/science/sciencenow/la-sci-sn-get-up-20140731-story.html

[12] Kessler RC, Chiu WT, Demler O, Walters EE. Prevalence, severity, and comorbidity of twelve-month DSM-IV disorders in the National Comorbidity Survey Replication (NCS-R). Archives of General Psychiatry, 2005 Jun;62(6):617-27.

is to try to make it go away—immediately if at all possible. The last thing we want to do is sit with our fear, anger, insecurity, confusion, regret, self-loathing, loneliness, or whatever else may be causing our distress. Unfortunately, we often just mask our symptoms, without addressing the underlying issue to which our souls may be trying to draw our attention.

Since 1980 I've devoted my professional life to helping patients deal effectively with addiction, bereavement, depression, post-traumatic stress, acute and chronic stress, and other health issues. I've seen the amount of suffering people are experiencing. I've seen what a ruin addiction can make of their lives—forcing them to wrestle with dark forces that—to them—seem overwhelming. Their agony is so intense that I doubt I could stay in this line of work if I didn't *know* from my clinical experience, which has been confirmed in over 1,500 individual cases, that there is an effective treatment that will bring them through their dark night of the soul. Moreover, it will restore their lives just like a reboot can restore your computer. It is my great joy and privilege to offer this treatment to my patients and to spread the word about it to you who are reading this book.

But first, let's look a bit more closely at this epidemic of addiction.

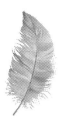

"Be kind whenever possible. It is always possible."
—Dalai Lama

CHAPTER THREE

Opiate Addiction: A Lethal Side-Effect of Pain Relief

One of my patients, Bruce, was addicted to opiates as a result of pain meds prescribed for a work-related accident. Unable to work, he was very concerned about his dependence for several reasons. First, his pain threshold had diminished as his tolerance for the pain meds increased. As a result, he needed more than the amount he was prescribed each month. Second, his family and former co-workers did not know he was addicted, but it was getting harder and harder to hide. As all opiate addicts know, when you run out of your meds you have limited options. You either doctor-shop for another prescription, find a source for buying opiates on the street to keep the withdrawal symptoms at bay, or you simply go through the hell of withdrawal. Bruce was now at the place where he could only buy his medication on the street. He was living on savings, which were quickly dwindling. His wife was asking him where the money was going, and he had to lie to her, which created more guilt and shame.

Until his accident and subsequent addiction, Bruce had been an exemplary "all-American" husband and father: coaching his kids' soccer teams, attending their school events, and taking summer vacations with his entire extended family—including his parents, sisters, and brothers. He was a deacon at his church, which he attended every Sunday. He had a strong family and community support system, but no one knew his secret. The good news for Bruce was that he was very healthy, save for the physical pain he suffered due to the accident and subsequent surgery. He was now suffering mental pain because he had become someone even *he* didn't recognize. He was short-tempered, didn't sleep well, was irritable with his wife, had lost confidence in being able to provide for his family, had decreased energy, was confused and foggy in his thinking, plus had the dreadful guilt and shame he felt about it all.

We talked at length, and I tried my best to help him understand that I knew he hadn't set out to become addicted, and that I also knew he didn't become addicted because he liked "to party." Many people become addicted from circumstance, not choice. In fact, I have yet to meet a person who chose to be addicted. Some fall prey to it innocently by taking prescribed medications to excess unwittingly. Some are too young to believe the truth that alcohol and drugs hijack your brain; some just want to "fit in" or "be cool," believing that addiction won't happen to them. But without exception, once the dependence vice tightened its grip they were trapped.

When I told him that we could stop the cravings with minimal withdrawal in 10 short days, he said, "Where do I sign?" It wasn't until he asked what the cost would be that I saw the tears rising in his eyes. He apologized for taking up my time but said he couldn't afford it. Then he looked at me and began taking off his watch, asking, "Would you be willing to take my watch for payment?" That was when *my* tears surfaced. I told him to put his watch back on because we would find a way. We worked out a payment plan because I was certain that he would be able to pay once he got back to work following the treatment.

I walked him to the door, where he turned and whispered "thank you" before hugging me goodbye.

The rise in both acute and chronic pain rates in the U.S. has led to a skyrocketing increase in prescriptions for opioid pain relievers like hydrocodone (e.g., Vicodin), oxycodone (e.g., OxyContin and Percocet), morphine (e.g., Kadian, Avinza), codeine, and related drugs. The National Institute on Drug Abuse (NIDA) reports that the number of prescriptions for opiates has risen nearly threefold since 1991: from 76 million to 210 million in 2010. NIDA further estimates that the percentage of individuals prescribed an opiate pain reliever who will become addicted ranges from 3% to 40%. One NIDA-reported study narrowed the range to 23%.[13] Physicians who try to reduce the risk of addiction by restricting the numbers of prescriptions they fill for the same patient have, inadvertently, driven people to heroin, which is a lot less costly to buy illegally than a prescription opiate.

Opiates work by attaching to opioid receptors in the brain, spinal cord, and various organs and, as a result, reduce the number and intensity of pain messages sent to the brain and the corresponding feelings of pain in the patient. Opiates are very effective pain-relievers, particularly for severe pain; however, over time the body becomes habituated to their effect—meaning that a greater dose is required to deliver the same level of relief. Also, many persons become increasingly sensitized to pain. This is why these drugs are identified as habit-forming, addictive, and as a result, tightly regulated.

Despite this fact, society—and even the medical establishment—continues to refer to opiate addiction as indicative of a character defect. Even NIDA literature[14] draws a distinction

---

[13] National Institute on Drug Abuse. (2014). Drug Facts: Heroin. Bethesda, MD: National Institute on Drug Abuse. Available at http://www.drugabuse.gov/publications/drugfacts/heroin.

[14] https://www.drugabuse.gov/sites/default/files/rrprescription.pdf

between "dependence—the body's *normal* adaptations to chronic exposure to a drug" and addiction, which, NIDA claims, "is distinguished by compulsive drug seeking and use despite sometimes devastating consequences." This is an affront to the accepted classification of addiction as a disease and minimizes the imperative of physical dependence. No one engages in "compulsive drug seeking despite devastating consequences" without an overwhelming dictate by the body to get it what it needs. This is the very definition of addiction: a condition of physical dependence created by rising drug tolerance and increased pain sensitivity. In fact, NIDA notes that "In either case, withdrawal symptoms may occur if drug use is suddenly reduced or stopped. These symptoms can include restlessness, muscle and bone pain, insomnia, diarrhea, vomiting, cold flashes with goose bumps ("cold turkey"), and involuntary leg movements." (ibid)

Taken as prescribed, opioids can be used to manage pain safely and effectively. However, when taken beyond the bounds of prescribed use, even a single large dose can cause severe respiratory depression and death. The American Association of Addiction Medicine (ASAM) reports that "Drug overdose is the leading cause of accidental death in the US—more than traffic accidents, falls, drownings, fires, and accidental shootings—with 47,055 lethal drug overdoses in 2014. Opioid addiction is driving this epidemic, with 18,893 overdose deaths related to prescription pain relievers, and 10,574 overdose deaths related to heroin in 2014.[15] ASAM further reports that, from 1999 to 2008, overdose death rates, sales and substance use disorder treatment admissions related to prescription pain relievers increased in parallel. The overdose death rate in 2008 was nearly four times the 1999 rate. Sales of prescription pain relievers in 2010

---

[15] http://www.asam.org/docs/default-source/advocacy/opioid-addiction-disease-facts-figures.pdf

were four times those in 1999, and the substance use disorder treatment admission rate in 2009 was six times the 1999 rate.

NIDA reports that in 2007, the number of overdose deaths from prescription opioids outnumbered deaths from heroin and cocaine combined. And the skyrocketing number of opioid prescriptions has fueled heroin addiction and overdose rates, too. Four in five new heroin users started out misusing prescription painkillers.[16] And a whopping 94% of respondents in a 2014 survey of people in treatment for opioid addiction said they chose to use heroin because prescription opioids were "far more expensive and harder to obtain."[17]

Tragically, persons who have been through rehab and broken their addiction are at greater risk of overdose should they relapse. Not realizing that their body no longer requires—or can withstand—the doses they were taking prior to withdrawal, they all too often go into respiratory failure or cardiac arrest on a single dose.[18]

[16] Jones CM. Heroin use and heroin use risk behaviors among nonmedical users of prescription opioid pain relievers - United States, 2002-2004 and 2008-2010. Drug Alcohol Depend. 2013 Sep 1;132(1-2):95- 100. doi: 10.1016/j.drugalcdep.2013.01.007. Epub 2013 Feb 12

[17] Cicero TJ, Ellis MS, Surratt HL, Kurtz SP. The changing face of heroin use in the United States: a retrospective analysis of the past 50 years. JAMA Psychiatry. 2014;71(7):821-826. 10 National Institute of Drug Abuse. (2015). Drug Facts: Prescription and Over-the-Counter Medications. Bethesda, MD: National Institute of Drug Abuse. Available at http://www.drugabuse.gov/publications/drugfacts/prescription-over-counter-medications

[18] https://www.drugabuse.gov/about-nida/legislative-activities/testimony-to-congress/2016/americas-addiction-to-opioids-heroin-prescription-drug-abuse

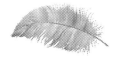

But what if I fail of my purpose here? It is but to keep the nerves at strain, to dry one's eyes and laugh at a fall, and baffled, get up and begin again.
—Robert Browning

CHAPTER FOUR

Synthetic Opioids: More Potent, More Deadly

Although heroin and Suboxone (a drug developed for opioid detox and maintenance therapies, theoretically to replace methadone) currently share the national opioid spotlight, a new and deadlier epidemic is on the horizon. Fentanyl, a synthetic opioid 50 times more powerful than heroin and 100 times the potency of morphine according to the CDC,[19] is traditionally used for acute care in emergency settings and breakthrough pain management for cancer patients. First branded by Janssen Pharmaceutical in 1960 as Sublimaze, a general anesthetic, fentanyl analogs such as carfentanil, sufentanil, alfentanil, and remifentanil are estimated to have as much as *10,000 times* the potency of morphine. [20]

By the 1990s, fentanyl was introduced by various generic makers branding the fentanyl patch, and the next decade brought innovations such as the fentanyl lollipop, a dissolving tablet, and a top-selling sublingual spray branded Subsys by

---

[19] https://www.cdc.gov/drugoverdose/data/fentanyl.html

[20] https://www.ncbi.nlm.nih.gov/pmc/articles/PMC4137794/; https://www.unodc.org/documents/scientific/Global_SMART_Update_17_web.pdf

Insys Pharma. As of 2013, fentanyl was the most widely used synthetic opioid in medicine.

The overwhelming majority of fentanyl seized by law enforcement is not diverted from pharmacies and hospitals; rather it is manufactured illegally. To date, more than 12 analogs of fentanyl have been produced clandestinely and identified in the U.S. DEA investigations point to sources in China and Mexico as the global manufacturers and suppliers of fentanyl. Raw materials and chemicals sold from Chinese warehouses, as well as machinery to make the pills, have been seized by the DEA. Mexican cartels have discovered fentanyl is more efficient and less expensive to produce than heroin. Heroin production requires farming, harvesting, processing paste, packaging, transport, and manpower, whereas fentanyl only requires chemical material and precursors to make the drug, *or* the finished product can be purchased directly from Chinese manufacturers. Russ Baer, a DEA spokesman quoted in Vice.com, clearly articulates the economic advantages for organized crime of fentanyl over heroin: "A kilo of heroin sells in the U.S. for $60,000, with a street value of several hundred thousand dollars when diluted and sold by the gram. A kilo of fentanyl can be produced for $4000-$6000 and, with its extreme potency, it can be cut into 24 kilos yielding a profit of $1.3 million."[21]

The DEA calls the spread of fentanyl and its analogs "an unprecedented threat," due not only to the rapid growth of their use but their stratospheric death toll. A May 2017 Pew Foundation article cites round numbers for fentanyl overdoses: In 2014, the drug killed more than 5,000 Americans according to the Centers for Disease Control and Prevention. The next year nearly 10,000 Americans died from fentanyl-related overdoses, or 30% of the 33,000 opioid deaths in 2015.[22] Commenting on

---

[21] https://news.vice.com/article/americas-new-deadliest-drug-fentanyl)

[22] (http://www.pewtrusts.org/en/research-and-analysis/blogs/stateline/2017/05/08/as-fentanyl-spreads-states-step-up-responses

fentanyl's rapid penetration and resulting overdose statistics, Robert Anderson, who oversees death statistics at the Centers for Disease Control and Prevention remarked, "I don't think we've ever seen anything like this.... certainly, not in modern times." Andrea Walker, director of behavioral health services, Frederick County, Maryland, an epicenter of fentanyl overdoses, added, "If death were a deterrent to drug use, we wouldn't be in this situation. But that's not the way addiction works. The disease reprograms the brain to seek more drugs, even in the face of death." (ibid)

Non-medical use of fentanyl by individuals without opiate tolerance is very dangerous, and even those with opiate tolerances are at high risk for overdose because, once the fentanyl is in the user's system, it is extremely difficult to stop the course of its absorption. Intravenous fentanyl addicts report immediate euphoria and paralysis in the arms and chest the instant the drug is injected. Consequently, most overdose victims are discovered with the needle still intravenous.

Fentanyl powder has frequently been used by dealers to increase potency or compensate for low-quality heroin. Traci Green, an epidemiologist and deputy director of the Injury Prevention Center at Boston Medical Center, explains that on the West Coast heroin is black tar. But eastern states trade a white powder variety, in which fentanyl is easily (and imprecisely) mixed, causing confusion for users (and a plausible explanation for its origins in New England). The consequences can be tragic. "The margin of error is very small with fentanyl," Green said.

CDC Investigator Matthew Gladden offers more insight into fentanyl overdose, suggesting that people were likely dying because they were taking fentanyl unknowingly, both in cut heroin or counterfeit pills made to look like OxyContin and other sought-after brands. In Florida, pills that look like oxycodone, Percocet, or Xanax have been recovered and found to be fentanyl, and are responsible for a string of deaths. A 2016

CNN story reported on fentanyl pills labeled NORCO, identical to generic hydrocodone, which were responsible for 30 deaths within 72 hours in Sacramento.[23]

Perhaps the most famous case of counterfeit fentanyl overdose was the tragic passing of pop sensation Prince. The Midwest Coroner's Office found that Prince died of fentanyl toxicity, and law enforcement officials recovered pills at Paisley Park Studio identified as hydrocodone that were actually fentanyl.

Another synthetic even more deadly than fentanyl has emerged in U.S. drug trade. Carfentanil, an analog of fentanyl, was first synthesized by Janssen Pharma in 1974 and branded Wildnil. The *American Journal of Emergency Medicine* claims Wildnil (carfentanil) has 10,000 times the potency of morphine and is only approved for use by veterinarians as a tranquilizing agent to rapidly incapacitate large animals, such as elephants. Because of its potency, hospitals rarely use carfentanil in laboratory settings and veterinarians who handle the drug wear protective gloves, masks, and aprons, as it can be lethal even when absorbed through the skin. To date, carfentanil is the most powerful commercial opioid.

At Springfield Wellness Center, we've treated some patients who were addicted to synthetic opioids, including fentanyl. Most are also simultaneously addicted to other opiate painkillers, prescribed to help them deal with excruciating pain. While we understand the value of painkillers in these terrible circumstances, the problem is that long-term use of narcotic painkillers decreases the body's production of its own painkillers, the endorphins. Patients with chronic pain develop tolerance to the drug or drugs, become addicted, and then, when cut off, are left with even worse pain.

One young woman came to us after a serious accident that had broken her neck and a half-dozen other bones in her body.

---

[23] http://www.cnn.com/2016/04/05/health/sacramento-overdoses-and-deaths/index.html)

She'd been partially paralyzed for months and, though she had regained the use of her legs, was in such terrible, constant pain that she'd been prescribed four opioid pain relievers, including opana, and had become addicted. She was an absolute sweetheart. When she came to us, I'd sit at her side, hold her hand, and try to comfort her to the best of my ability. I rarely left her side. We connected as strongly as if she were my daughter.

In 10 short days of BR+NAD™ treatment, this young woman was free of all her cravings and withdrawal symptoms. That was cause enough for celebration. Better still, she was also free of her pain—a benefit often seen—*because her brain had been treated*. BR+NAD™ had given it a reboot. Her pain thresholds had returned to normal, presumably because her body's endorphin production had resumed and her pain receptors had improved.

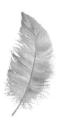

"We gain strength and courage, and confidence by each experience in which we really stop to look fear in the face…we must do that which we think we cannot."
—Eleanor Roosevelt

CHAPTER FIVE

Methamphetamines, Cocaine, Benzos, and Alcohol: A Fleeting Sense Of Well-Being And Control

Although methamphetamines are prescribed in limited circumstances, most typically for attention deficit, hyperactivity disorder (ADHD), their illicit use far exceeds their prescribed use. Highly addictive, methamphetamine (also called meth, crystal, crystal meth, chalk, crank, ice, and other street names) is similar chemically to amphetamine: a white, odorless, bitter-tasting crystalline powder. It can be taken orally, smoked, snorted, or dissolved in water or alcohol and injected. Smoking or injecting the drug delivers it very quickly to the brain, where it produces an immediate, intense euphoria. Because the pleasure also fades quickly, users often take repeated doses, trying to maintain the high.

Methamphetamines work by increasing the brain's supply of dopamine—the neurotransmitter of reward, pleasure, motivation, and motor function. As a result, meth produces a euphoric feeling of invincibility—like there's nothing the user cannot do.

Not surprisingly, it has become a popular drug for marginalized people—laid off, unemployed, perhaps uneducated—who feel that life offers them few prospects for success.

Unfortunately, chronic methamphetamine use has many disastrous health consequences, including anxiety, confusion, insomnia, mood problems, violent behavior, paranoia, hallucinations, delusions, extreme weight loss, severe dental problems ("meth mouth"), skin sores caused by scratching, overdose, and early death. It also increases the risk of contracting infectious diseases like HIV and hepatitis B and C because the feelings of invincibility that accompany its use undermine the caution that normally keeps people from sharing needles or engaging in unprotected sex. Meth use also masks the effects of alcohol, increasing the risk of alcohol poisoning. There is also evidence that methamphetamine use speeds the progression of HIV/AIDS and its consequences.

Although the National Institute on Drug Abuse claims "There are no FDA-approved medications to treat methamphetamine addiction,"[24] I can confirm that there is a natural treatment that is effective in treating meth addiction—a result I have witnessed hundreds of times. As I've said, it is called BR+NAD™ and it is a simple coenzyme of niacin.

If you asked me which addictive substance was the most frightening—crack cocaine or methamphetamine—I would be hard-pressed to choose. All addictive substances have the potential to hijack the human mind and body when taken in large doses, but I know that crack and meth dominate the "fast lane to addiction." Addictions to these two substances share some of the same side effects and adversely affect a person in lightning speed. Both are strong central nervous system stimulants used primarily as a recreational drug. Both are euphoriant and neurotoxic to the dopaminergic neurons of the human midbrain.

---

[24] https://www.drugabuse.gov/drugs-abuse/commonly-abused-drugs-charts#meth

The initial attraction to using crack or meth, generally in low doses, is to increase alertness, concentration, and energy, while reducing appetite for weight loss. When taken in higher doses, which generally occurs as tolerance develops with repeated use, the drugs can cause rapid mood swings, induced psychosis—including hallucinations, delusions, and paranoia—and even violence. The drugs also have extremely deleterious physical effects, as noted previously. Perhaps worst of all, while other addictions take hold after repeated use, addiction to these two substances can occur on first use.

Why would anyone try either of these drugs for fun? We don't know, and they don't know! My lame fallback position is that "addiction defies logic." There are as many variables involved in addiction as there are differences in thumbprints. Genetics, epigenetics, and oxidative stress all play a role, and each combination of factors is unique to each human walking the earth. We can also analyze the psycho-social-spiritual elements and come up with different explanations as to why some individuals try and become addicted to these substances and others don't. I could spend pages on suggestions of how to address this topic based on my experience as a therapist. Instead, let me give you three examples of patients we have treated.

One was a kind, timid woman who had dropped out of high school and found herself in the grip of methamphetamine. Her husband loved her and was willing to do everything he could to help her. He was well-meaning, but did what so many significant others do with their addicted family members: he shamed her, scared her, threatened to leave her, and blamed her for being weak. He didn't understand why she couldn't control herself and just stay away from the people who would give the drug to her. In one session following a relapse, I asked him to give me his pack of cigarettes. I asked him if he would not smoke until our next scheduled session a week later as a way to support his wife. He would control his addiction, and she would control hers.

Guess who had a pack of cigarettes in his pocket a week later? Fortunately, this sweet woman was given a second chance thanks to BR+NAD™ treatment. Last, I heard she was doing very well.

Another patient was a very successful businessman who had everything going for him. His wife, too, was a successful professional and his children were good athletes and successful students. When meeting him, you would never guess he was addicted to crack. His life became consumed by the addiction, costing him his businesses. He filed for bankruptcy and was fortunate enough to keep his family together because of his wife's devotion and his love for his children. After 10 days on the BR+NAD™ treatment, he was able to break his chemical addiction, but it was necessary for him to go to a residential program for follow-up care. In some cases, a person needs residential treatment to minimize stressful influences. Upon his return, he was able to resume managing his businesses with his family intact.

The most challenging case I have ever worked with was an entire family addicted to meth. The husband, wife, and children were all addicted. This was a near-hopeless situation. Without establishing and designating a remote town a sober living community (which has been a fantasy of mine), very little can be done to help a family of addicts. Each member needs to be separated from the others for an extended period. Unfortunately, this solution requires significant financial backing not available to most families struggling with addiction.

Because the members of this family all lived together, if one relapsed, they all relapsed, perpetuating the cycle. All of them completed the intravenous (IV) BR+NAD™ treatment, and each got a good response, but their individual post-acute withdrawal symptoms (PAWS) showed up at different times, and before long they all had relapsed and were using again…together!

Theirs is one of the saddest stories of all my years of therapeutic practice. I care deeply for each member of this family. We spent a great deal of time fighting the meth monster together, to no avail. I still think of them often and would like to know how they are doing today, but I'm afraid to make the call.

When I look for a common denominator in cases like these, I find a history of trouble in school, academically and/or behaviorally. They start drinking alcohol or smoking at an early age; they report growing up with verbal and/or physical abuse from one or both parents; they no longer practice their faith or go to church, nor claim to have any spiritual connections, and they each have financial resources that support their addiction. These similarities help reveal why, though addiction itself is a brain disease that responds to BR+NAD™ treatment, a more comprehensive therapeutic approach is often needed to address all of the issues that have led to addiction.

Central Nervous System (CNS) depressants

Benzodiazepines—Xanax, Valium, and others—are a class of depressants that affect the central nervous system and are frequently prescribed as a sedative, muscle relaxant, anticonvulsant, or hypnotic to treat panic and anxiety disorders, insomnia, migraines, seizures, restless leg syndrome, Tourette syndrome, and epilepsy. People are often surprised to learn that anxiety disorders are the most common mental illness in the U.S.—affecting 40 million adults in the United States age 18 and older, or 18% of the population.[25]

Benzodiazepines are powerfully addictive, however, and because of their prevalence as a prescription medication are among the most abused drugs in the country. Although "abuse" is defined as anything other than the prescribed dosage,

---

[25] https://www.nimh.nih.gov/health/statistics/prevalence/any-anxiety-disorder-among-adults.shtml

benzodiazepines can also be injected or snorted. Two "benzos" in particular—Xanax and Valium—are well-known by their proprietary names. Other names for benzos include bennies, downers, tranks, vals, sleepers, moggies, and more.

Benzodiazepines work by enhancing the activity of the neurotransmitter GABA (Gamma Amino Butyric Acid), which is the brain's major inhibitory transmitter. A central nervous system depressant, GABA's function is to slow things down. For nervous systems in an agitated or hypervigilant state, this is experienced as calming.

Long-term use of benzodiazepines, however, can result in dependency or addiction, with debilitating side effects that include delirium, dry heaves, hallucinations, impaired coordination, increased risk of suicide, seizures, slurred speech, vertigo, and "paradoxical effects," which magnify the symptoms the drug was prescribed to treat. A person prescribed Valium to relieve anxiety, for example, may instead experience an intense panic attack. A patient taking benzos to relieve pain may instead find their pain magnified. Benzodiazepines are often taken with other drugs, including alcohol, marijuana, amphetamines, and methamphetamines, and opiates, either prescribed or illicit, which complicates recovery. Symptoms of benzodiazepine overdose include drowsiness, confusion, dizziness, blurred vision, weakness, slurred speech, lack of coordination, and difficulty breathing. In the worst-case scenario, respiratory depression can be fatal.

At Springfield Wellness Center, we've successfully treated scores of people for benzo addiction. Two, in particular, come to mind. One was a young mother from North Dakota who'd become addicted after being prescribed benzodiazepines for her chronic, acute anxiety. She had two young children and didn't want anyone to know she was addicted—which is why she'd come to an out-of-state clinic. She was very frightened, as well as desperate, because she doubted we'd be able to help her. In fact, it took 12 days of treatment because at the time we didn't have Archway Apothecary as our NAD+ provider. I'll have more to say later about the powerful difference Archway has made in our treatment efficacy. For now, it's enough to know that Archway found a way to formulate NAD+ without heat— which results in a purer, higher potency form of the product— which means our patients benefit that much faster.

At any rate, we sent this woman home, free of the drug, withdrawal symptoms, and cravings, and I never heard from her again until, four years later, I got a Christmas card showing a photo of two handsome young boys—her sons. The note said simply, "Thank you. I'm free." That was a wonderful Christmas bonus.

More recently, we treated a woman who was a successful theater professional when Hurricane Katrina hit. She evacuated with her mother, but the experience left her shaken to the point of PTSD. A few months later her mother died; then her husband divorced her. By the time she came to us, she was too fearful to leave the house or even get up off the sofa.

A friend brought her in for assessment, and the woman was so agitated she couldn't sit still for more than 30 seconds. She kept jumping up saying, "I can't do it; I'm not going to be able to do it." I kept telling her, slowly, that if she completed our program, she would never have to feel like this again. She finally agreed, and it took her just a few days to get through withdrawal from the benzos. Then she entered the happy, euphoric stage of BR+NAD™ treatment—where clients are so thrilled to feel good again they can't stop grinning, laughing, and bubbling over with enthusiasm. One day she looked outside at a pond on our property and said to me, "You know, I think I'd like to walk around that pond."

"By yourself?" I asked. "Well go on! Of course, you can!"

She did and afterward went home to resume her life. Sadly, today this patient is not doing well after years of sobriety. The stressful events of her life became overwhelming once again and the doctor she was seeing put her back on the medication that brought her to us in the first place. She couldn't afford the long-term residential care she needed to resolve the new stress that was consuming her life.

Alcohol

Alcohol is by far the most commonly abused drug in the United States, with 16 million adults counted as having an "alcohol use disorder," or AUD. Although it is far more socially acceptable than any of the other drugs to which Americans are addicted, excessive alcohol consumption, either on occasion, or chronically, has serious negative health effects. For starters, alcohol interferes with the brain's communication pathways, disrupting mood and behavior and making it harder to think clearly and move with coordination. Chronic over-consumption of alcohol can damage the heart, causing cardiomyopathy – stretching and drooping of the heart muscle; arrhythmias – irregular heartbeats; stroke; and high blood pressure. Long-term alcohol consumption also stresses—and can permanently damage—the liver, leading to unhealthy fat deposits, alcoholic hepatitis, fibrosis, and cirrhosis—all of which impair liver functioning. Alcohol consumption also causes the pancreas to produce toxic substances that can eventually lead to pancreatitis, a dangerous inflammation and swelling of the blood vessels in the pancreas that prevents proper digestion. Drinking to excess can also increase the risk of developing cancers of the mouth, esophagus, throat, liver, breast, and immune system. Overall, excessive alcohol consumption can weaken the immune system, making the body more susceptible to all kinds of disease. Chronic drinkers are more liable to contract diseases like pneumonia and tuberculosis than people who do not drink much.[26] And of course, driving under the influence of alcohol is a major cause of traffic accidents and fatalities—ending the lives of some 10,000 people annually.[27]

New Orleans, where I've lived most of my life, has a culture that encourages drinking—and early drinking. One of its nicknames is "The City That Care Forgot," but in truth, many people forget their cares because they're wasted. Of course, their cares are waiting for them when they sober up.

One client, Evan, was part of a large Catholic family. He had begun drinking at an early age and then started combining opiates with his alcohol. The combination applied the fatal blow to his marriage, although his wife was still physically present. Sensing her emotional distance, however, sent Evan deeper into addiction until his brother brought him in for treatment. Everything about him shouted the rage he was carrying inside. Even the shirt he wore reflected his wrath. It was painted with a cobra on the front, coiled and ready to strike, mouth open, exposing the fangs.

Evan went through treatment and transformed into one of the sweetest young men I'd ever experienced. He went home clean. I heard later that his wife left him...and then I stopped hearing from him. It's not the role of a therapist to chase a patient, so I simply waited. Three years later I got a frantic phone call from a woman who said her boyfriend was in trouble, violent, sick, but wouldn't go to the ER. The only person he'd talk to was Paula Norris.

I told the woman to bring him in, and Evan was indeed in very bad shape. He had to be helped out of the car and into the

[26] https://www.niaaa.nih.gov/alcohol-health/alcohols-effects-body
[27] Department of Transportation (US), National Highway Traffic Safety Administration (NHTSA). Traffic Safety Facts 2014 data: alcohol-impaired driving. Washington, DC: NHTSA; 2015 [cited 2016 Feb 5]

clinic; he couldn't walk or talk or focus very well. My staff was scared; he needed to be in the emergency room. I took the two into my office for privacy and tried unsuccessfully to find out what Evan had taken. The longer we talked, the more Evan began to slide down the sofa, unable to speak clearly.

Since he couldn't tell me what he had taken, I told him it was going to be necessary for him to go to the emergency room. He refused to go until I agreed to go with them. It was my first introduction to how addictive patients are treated by some ER medical staff. The "helping" professionals I witnessed that day were lacking in empathic care. They certainly were skilled in handling his medical needs, but their disdain was thinly veiled. I stayed until Evan was stable and discharged. I insisted that he come to the clinic the next morning by 8:00 A.M. to begin the second round of BR+NAD™ treatment. The next day he arrived on time, which often signifies a sincere desire to get better.

My new nurses were nervous; they'd seen what he'd been like the day before. But I told them to trust the process and wait to see the person who'd emerge after a couple of days of BR+NAD™ treatment. They saw for themselves how effective the treatment is.

This story has a surprising ending. Evan was relationship-phobic following his divorce, so his girlfriend, the woman who called me on that fateful day, requested that they engage in couple's counseling as part of Evan's aftercare plan. I saw them for several months. Once I realized that Evan was depressed, I referred him to Dr. Mestayer for possible medication. The medication prescribed was Wellbutrin, which was very helpful, so we were able to discontinue the counseling.

Wedding bells were ringing; I was no longer needed. We kept in touch over the years and, not long ago Evan contacted me after he heard a radio advertisement for Springfield Wellness Center. He sent me a picture of his 2004 Treatment Graduation Diploma, a picture of his Twenty-four Hours a Day meditation book, and a picture of the last page in the book with a text that said," I was going through my file cabinet the other day and found this. The little black book I still read every day and at the end of every year I make a mark to keep count of my years of sobriety. (14 marks so far) I am living proof that the treatment you do does work! Tell Dr. Mestayer I said hello. Love you both for saving my life." Evan is happily married and doing very well with his business, too. I smile inside as I write his story.

Another patient, Keith, age 62, had suffered from alcoholism since ninth grade and had completed various in-patient treatment programs, sometimes able to stay sober for years at a time. "But I was miserable every day," he said. "I felt like I was locked away inside and could never get out. So, I'd always start drinking again." After spending "a year drunk on the couch," his wife drove him to Springfield Wellness Center. By the time he arrived, he was so weak he had to be helped up the steps. Once inside, I began taking his history, learning what had brought him to this extremely depleted condition, and telling him what I believed we could do for him. He presented as a disheveled retired science teacher and Vietnam veteran. He wore a tattered t-shirt, shorts that exposed his swollen legs, and flip-flops. I was sure an attractive man was underneath the long hair and beard that covered his face. At first glance, I thought he was intoxicated, but I was wrong. He was simply extremely weak from the daily bottles of whiskey he had been consuming since his retirement. His wife had moved out of the house but would check on him from time to time to make sure he had food. She could not handle watching him "give up" or "give in" to his addiction to alcohol. Keith, at one point in his life, had been sober for 13 years, which he described as the most miserable years of his life.

Later he admitted, "I thought you were telling me all kinds of witch-doctor stuff to get my money." Then he said, "But after the first treatment, I was finally born. Not 'reborn.' The person who is me finally came out. For the first time in 62 years, I like who I am."

After the 10-day detox treatment, Keith saw me for counseling once a week for several months. He was doing very well, enjoying his hobbies and his love for the game of golf. He was able to structure his time to support his improved health. I told the nurses once that, "When Keith shows up with a haircut and shaven face, I will know he is well." Not long after I made that statement, I heard one of the nurses call me, in a very excited tone, "Come see." I walked over to meet the man at the door but didn't recognize Keith until I got close enough to hug him. All I said to him was, "I *knew* there was a handsome man under all that hair!"

Of course, people with a dependence on one drug, are often dependent—if not outright addicted—to more than one. If it takes half a bottle of alcohol and a couple of benzos to enable you to sleep through the night, for example, you're likely to need a pretty robust stimulant to jumpstart you again in the morning.

Freddy was one of our tough cases. He was an honor student and athlete in Delaware until he was falsely accused by a fellow student of an egregious infraction. The principal expelled him, which was the beginning of a negative spiral that led to drugs, alcohol, nightmares, anxiety, self-loathing, lack of purpose, fatigue, loss of friendships, and family discord. His parents brought him to Springfield Wellness Center after several failed attempts to help their son. His mother clearly believed that the expulsion from school was traumatic enough to cause PTS, to which addiction to opiates and benzos had been added.

As fate would have it, we were able to heal that triggering trauma—as well as free him from addiction—when Freddy was falsely accused of something at the clinic. This time, however, the event was redemptive. Another patient successfully defended Freddy and the "principal" at Springfield didn't expel him. The truth was revealed and we believed him! That allowed a strong, cathartic release of tears that helped wash away the pain he had carried for so many years.

I developed a strong therapeutic alliance with Freddy and to this day he continues to text me updates on his challenges and successes with school and relationships. It has been over a year since his treatment, and he is preparing for an internship in counseling psychology to complete his master's degree. There have been no slips or relapses during the year. Freddy has a goal and a purpose! He is self-disciplined and has followed through with every one of the actions we agreed upon in his aftercare plan. He has experienced disappointments at school, but he has been able to resist any temptation to "give up." He has stayed on the path of his own recovery. He will be one of the first of the next generation of mental health professionals who will know the value of BR+NAD™!

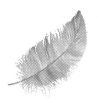

You leave old habits behind by starting out with the thought, 'I release the need for this in my life.'
—Wayne Dyer

Kim's story

Kim came to us because she realized she was drinking too much. She thought she had it under control until one day she realized that both her mother and daughter, whom she loves dearly, were concerned about her behavior. She wouldn't return their calls in the evening because she didn't want them to hear her voice or ask her questions, which would tip them off that she had been drinking. When she came to us, she wanted to keep a low profile and not let anyone know she'd come for treatment. She turned out to be one of the lucky ones who got the "eraser effect" with one treatment—no lingering feeling that she'd like a drink, or even the sense that she'd ever "been a drinker." This is an effect that we still cannot adequately explain.

Kim credits a visit to John of God, or Joao de Deus, in Brazil a few months prior to her visit to Springfield Wellness Center with her remarkable recovery. John of God, considered the Miracle Man of Brazil, is an international healing medium who is quoted as proclaiming, "I do not cure anybody. God heals and in his infinite goodness permits the Entities to heal and console my brothers. I am merely an instrument in God's hands." As Kim says, she decided to go to Brazil to see John of God and deliver to him a note with her one prayer, which was to have alcohol removed from her life. Shortly after returning to the U.S., Kim found out about Springfield Wellness Center and made her fateful drive to her liberation.

Kim and her husband, Charles, had the treatment and both are approaching their sixth year of sobriety. I think that the way they implemented their aftercare plan has a lot to do with their outcome. They exercise regularly, eat well, meditate daily, and support each other in their personal growth. Kim is famous for "leading with love rather than fear," and she seems to have mastered it.

Their efforts to work with the local sheriff and district attorney in collaboration with us on a pilot project were very helpful and instructive. One of the five patients who participated was a young woman addicted to heroin. She had a very poor prognosis due to her drug history, but she had one very important companion who did not let her out of her sight (literally) during the treatment: her mother! She also had an advocate in Kim, who supported her throughout the BR+NAD™ detox and the 90-day residential program that followed. That young woman called today to thank Kim for helping her with her addiction recovery and wanted Kim to know that today was her two-year anniversary of sobriety.

Kim no longer wishes to hide her story, which she is committed to using to help as many people as possible free themselves from the guilt and shame of addiction.

BR+NAD™ and Prison Reform

Now that there is serious bipartisan attention being given to prison reform, I'd like to suggest a unique but very effective addition to the First Step Act, which is designed to expand much-needed rehabilitation opportunities, while reducing mandatory minimum sentences for drug crimes. The intention is to reduce recidivism and facilitate a more promising re-entry opportunity into society.

What I propose is born out of 20 years of observation that BR+NAD™ Brain Restoration Treatment can significantly change the personality, temperament, confidence, kindness, and perceptions of individuals whose brains have been hijacked by substance abuse. I have seen this transformation in hundreds of cases, but the most dramatic transformation was a man who walked into Springfield Wellness Center as a "Skinhead" and in 10 little days walked out a "gentleman."

Had I not been a witness to these remarkable transformations,

I would not have begun to think of ways to help the inmates in prison for drug-related crimes. We all know what those crimes look like. Some are violent, some are not. They all cause harm. Lives are destroyed; families are destroyed; communities are destroyed. We, as a nation, have not yet found a solution to this scourge but I believe the First Step Act is a big first step in the right direction. I strongly believe—in fact, I *know*—that what I am going to suggest will enable the most successful outcomes for "First Step." It will give drug-addicted inmates their best chance of beating their addiction and overcoming their past criminal behavior by healing their brains. When the brain is healed, a person has the clarity of mind, confidence and motivation to succeed. It is wonderful to witness what having hope in your heart will do to promote success.

Here is the proposal in a nutshell:

1. Take a population of non-violent offenders who are incarcerated due to drug offenses and separate them from the general population. Move them to a part of the prison away from the violent or aggressive population.
2. Give them the 10-day protocol of the BR+NAD™ intravenous infusion, followed by monthly boosters consisting of one half-day infusion. Give vitamins, minerals, and BR+NAD supplements daily, as needed.
3. Provide weekly counseling sessions (individual, group and family), as well as daily meditation and Saturday or Sunday spiritual observance of their choice. Daily exercise and good nutrition will also enhance successful outcomes. Adding these to the "First Step" proposal will boost the positive outcomes we all are looking for.

There is a reason so many patients report that they started using again the day they were discharged from rehab. Addiction is first a brain disease and if the brain is not restored the patient, though "clean," is left with cravings and post-acute withdrawal syndrome (PAWS). BR+NAD™ treatment has proven to block craving and manage PAWS.

The success we have at Springfield Wellness Center is because we first address restoring the brain. Once the brain begins to clear up from the toxic pollutants that have hijacked it and the mid-brain defect is repaired you will have a person motived to succeed.

Once this trial population has demonstrated the success of my proposal, we could expand it to all non-violent drug offenders. To those who cry, "What about the cost?!" I answer, "The cost would be *far, far less* than the cost of repeated incarceration—to say nothing of the tragic loss of human potential, family ties, and community relationships.

Multiple addictions

As you may have noticed, many patients come to us with addictions to more than one substance. Although this compounds addiction's deleterious effects on one's health, it *does not reduce the effectiveness* of the treatment upon which I have based my career and professional reputation; the treatment to which I have devoted the past 20 years of my life and plan to devote whatever years are left to me. But first, let me tell you how addiction very nearly took my beloved daughter.

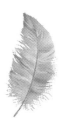

I have always believed…that whatever good or bad fortune may come our way we can always give it meaning and transform it into something of value.
—Hermann Hesse

CHAPTER SIX

The Cultural Becomes Personal

As a therapist, I'd worked for years with hundreds of patients struggling with addiction, anxiety, depression, post-traumatic stress (PTS), and scores of other ailments. I'd helped them deal with the emotional, psychological, and spiritual pain that prompted them to medicate with drugs and alcohol. I saw how frequently reliance on pain or anxiety medications devolved into full-blown addictions. When that happened, I'd send my patients to detox, or rehab, to deal with the physical disease of addiction. I'd provide the emotional and psychological support they needed once they were "clean." Nothing in my training or experience prepared me to understand the physical connection—the breakdown in the brain—that characterizes addiction, depression, trauma, concussion, CTE, chronic pain, and even Parkinson's and Alzheimer's. Then addiction came into my home.

In 1998, my happy, bubbly teenage daughter suddenly exhibited such a personality change that I suspected she was using drugs—although I didn't know which drugs, or how heavily she was involved. Overnight she became angry and argumentative and eventually fell into a deep depression. A friend told me about an American doctor practicing in Tijuana, Mexico, who was getting "miraculous" results with what he called NTR—Neurotransmission Restoration—therapy. My husband, — Dr. Richard Mestayer, III, who for 20 years was the medical director at Ochsner Foundation Hospital's Stress Treatment and Behavior Health units—was appalled at the very idea of sending her for treatment to Mexico. But I called and spoke with the director—Dr. William Hitt—and liked what I heard about his intravenous NTR therapy, so we decided to give it a try.

Dr. William Hitt was controversial due to his fearless experimentation and research on treating a wide range of diseases. He reported success with addictions, autoimmune diseases, allergies and viruses by employing intravenous amino acid therapies for neurotransmitter rebalancing, and intravenous ozone therapies to kill viruses such as HIV and hepatitis C. Dr. Hitt's general vexation regarding modern medicine resulted in his establishing the Hitt Center in Tijuana, Mexico, outside the purview of the AMA and the U.S. federal government. Best known for its work in the field of addiction, we were told that the William Hitt Center was an outgrowth of a World Health Organization grant given to Dr. Hitt and Mexican psychiatrist Dr. Velazquez Suarez. The grant allowed Dr. Hitt to continue his pioneering work to detoxify, cleanse, and stop cravings in the brains of alcoholics and drug addicts.

The Hitt Center's detoxification protocol helped rebalance the neurotransmitters in the brain damaged by drug use. Closely resembling the DPN Therapy developed by Dr. Paul O'Halloren at Shick-Shadel Hospital in Seattle (see Chapter 11), the treatment was described as a rapid detox from alcohol, prescription, and illicit drugs. Hitt's treatment used no benzodiazepines or opiates to combat withdrawal symptoms and, over the years, boasted low rates of recidivism.

His center reported treating well-known celebrities, including bestselling authors, film producers, actors, comedians, musicians and film composers—in part because they could detox in relative anonymity in Mexico. Many U.S. physicians and pioneers in the health and food revolution were themselves ongoing patients at the clinic, and while it was operational, the Hitt Center was featured on BBC and the Discovery Channel.

Dr. Hitt treated my daughter for 10 days using his intravenous protocols, which he described as an amino acid supplements with vitamins, minerals and coenzymes. She came home clean and happy; her personality returned to the child I knew. She was thereafter the designated driver for her high school friends, graduated from college with a degree in history, and has been addiction-free and successful ever since. The only things left for my daughter are to manage her oxidative stress and make peace with her fear and anger, which are lifelong endeavors for all of us.

It is because of my personal experience as a mother concerned for her daughter that I can speak honestly to other mothers when they call, desperate to help their own children. If they cry on the phone, I tend to cry with them because we have shared this experience. I know in the depths of my being that addiction is not just a theory or a diagnosis or a moral failing. It is a serious, life-threatening disease that has infected almost every home and every corner of our culture.

By the time someone decides to take the "chance" to get BR+NAD™ treatment, even though what they have read, been told, heard on the radio, or seen on TV sounds too good to be true, it is because their *pain* is greater than their *fear*. They fear their situation is hopeless because nothing so far has worked for them. Most have been through numerous rehabs, have been in trouble with the law, have lost their jobs, their families, their purpose and self-esteem, and believe they are doomed to life as an addict or alcoholic, a "loser" who lies, steals, and is an unreliable, selfish, manipulator. They sit with me quietly in most cases, full of shame and guilt and hopelessness, to listen to what I have to say about how this treatment—intravenous BR+NAD™—is different from the other approaches they have tried unsuccessfully. We start by acknowledging that, yes, it does sound like it is too good to be true, but if they want to be free from the darkness that has consumed their lives, this *is* a way out.

I assure them that we do not judge or criticize them because their brain has been hijacked by a substance. I try to help them understand that the brain mediates all aspects of our behavior and if the light in the brain isn't on, they are not able to see things clearly. BR+NAD™ turns on the light. When that happens, they will be able to make better choices because they will see their past, their present, and their future with the light of love, not self-loathing. Having impulse control is a major advantage as we travel through life. When your brain is hijacked, there is NO impulse control. Your brain is your computer. If it has been hijacked by a virus, it is not going to work for you. BR+NAD™ will remove the virus and is neuroprotective, too, so you can keep your brain working optimally for you. You don't abuse your other devices, so why abuse the most important device you have been given…your brain!

In the years that followed my daughter's treatment by Dr. Hitt, I often referred clients struggling with addiction to his center for detox treatment, and he would refer his American patients—once detoxified—to me for psychotherapy and aftercare.

One young man who'd gone to Dr. Hitt for treatment and then came to me for aftercare had been part of a group of 10 highly successful stockbrokers who'd made too much money too young. Of the 10, he was the only one still alive. The others had overdosed, been killed in accidents, or met other early deaths as a result of their addictions. I sent him to AA as part of his aftercare, and they told him that the results he'd experienced in getting clean were impossible; they were "too good to be true" and he was just "setting himself up for relapse." This young man, who'd been raised a Catholic in New Orleans, has since earned a Ph.D. in theology and is the minister of a large Baptist church in Nashville, Tennessee. His recovery was not "too good to be true." Nor was Dr. Hitt's treatment "too good to be true" for the other patients I referred to him.

However, because many patients were reluctant or unable to go to Mexico for medical care, I began to consider opening my own clinic in Louisiana, my home. In 1998, the Discovery Channel did a program on various alternative treatments for drug addiction—including Dr. Hitt's clinic in Mexico. The program was shown in Europe but not in the U.S. When I learned of this and mentioned it to a friend who worked at New Orleans television station WDSU, she produced a two-part series on Dr. Hitt's treatment for addiction. The program aired in New Orleans in 2000.

With this kind of validation, in 2001, I asked Dr. Hitt what I needed to do to prove to him that I could treat people here in the States using his protocols. We worked out an arrangement by which I'd take an addicted patient's medical history and fax it to Dr. Hitt, and he'd advise our medical director and me on the recommended proprietary formula—which differed depending on whether the addiction was to alcohol, opiates, benzodiazepines, or amphetamines. Dr. Hitt also supplied the product we used.

I succeeded in opening my clinic, in Louisiana, delivering Dr. Hitt's intravenous therapy. Then Hurricane Katrina hit, and our home and clinic were severely damaged. In the years before we could fully recover, Dr. Hitt died. We dropped everything and flew to Mexico for his funeral. I wrote and delivered his eulogy at his final resting place at Monte Tabor Convent, home to the sisters of the Trinitarians of Mary.

We thought we were out of business—at least in the addiction detox department—but, as fate would have it, we had an ally in Dr. Hitt's clinic. Being a deeply spiritual woman, this ally knew we needed the proprietary formulas to continue Dr. Hitt's work. She also knew that Dr. Hitt had been loath to share them while he was alive, but now that he was deceased she wasn't sure what was the right thing to do. Finally, she went to confession and asked her priest whether it would be morally right for her to share the formulas with us. The priest asked whether doing so would ease human suffering. When she said, "Oh yes," the priest gave her his blessing—and she shared with us what she knew, revealing that NAD+ was a key ingredient. This was later confirmed by independent laboratory analysis.

Soon afterward we met Sam Camp, who introduced us to Archway Apothecary, which is the source of our 99.99% pure NAD+. The quality of the NAD+ is critical to the effectiveness of our protocols, which far exceed the results from NAD+ sourced elsewhere—as we know from our own experience. A former Tulane University football player, Sam's personality and demeanor are those of a confident, successful businessman with a heart full of love for his family, friends, and fellowman. A man of faith, he has taken many risks in life and triumphed over many challenges. He endeared himself forever to me when, at the end of our very first meeting he walked my husband and me to the door of his impressive facility, took my hand and held it gently saying, "I'm one of those people who doesn't believe we meet by accident." I smiled and replied, "I'm one of those people, too!"

My greatest treatment embarrassment

After Dr. Hitt's death, his clinic received a call from a woman in India looking for treatment for one of her family members. The clinic had to deliver the bad news that Dr. Hitt had recently died, whereupon the woman asked if there was anyone else Dr. Hitt trusted who could provide the treatment. The clinic referred the woman to us as the provider most trusted and experienced with Dr. Hitt's formulas.

This beautiful woman, whom I will call Diva, was a desperate mother looking for help for a family member. She convinced us to come to India to treat her family member privately. We agreed to come and were treated with the highest esteem, seeing India from a VIP perspective—unlike my first trip when I spent a month at an ashram in Mumbai, back when it was Bombay. The generosity showered upon us was enormous, which is partly why I feel embarrassed. We met our host's very impressive friends and family members, who embraced us with warm acceptance and trust. My husband was even given a medical treatment for his back, which was his most successful to date, eliminating his pain for nearly a year! We were introduced to a host of medical professionals who asked us to explain Dr. Hitt's intravenous treatment. We had not yet discovered that the key ingredient in Dr. Hitt's product was NAD+.

Diva's family member got a good response to our treatment, using Dr. Hitt's product, which was far inferior to the Archway product we now use. Had we known what we know now our treatment results would have been better. We kept in touch with Diva for a year or so once returning to the U.S. When we discovered the truth about our product, we called to let her know. We had just begun our relationship with Archway and, at the time, there was not a process that would allow us to ship to India. We apologized for being misinformed about the key ingredient in our treatment's effectiveness, which is nicotinamide adenine dinucleotide. I certainly hope Diva didn't suffer any embarrassment as a result.

We lost contact with Diva over the years. Life had other plans for each of us. Still, I hold Diva in my heart and hope she is well. She is a grandmother now and I know how deeply we can fall in love when that happens.

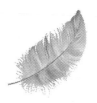

In the realm of ideas, everything depends on enthusiasm...
in the real world, all rests on perseverance.
—Johann Wolfgang von Goethe

CHAPTER SEVEN

What's So Special About NAD+?

NAD+ plays a crucial role in cell metabolism and repair. It is an important component of healthy mitochondrial functioning—the battery that powers our cells. Although the intravenous NAD+ therapies are relatively new, their evolution started over 100 years ago when the NAD+ coenzyme was discovered by British biochemists Arthur Harden and William John Young in 1906. NAD+ has been used for drug addiction rehabilitation in South Africa since the 1970s and was even used in the United States and Canada until it was abandoned— particularly for opiate addiction—in favor of methadone, and later Suboxone. Both methadone and suboxone, which could be taken orally—a less cumbersome and expensive way to administer treatment—though also addictive. (Cynics would say that both replacement drugs are also backed by Big Pharma, who has a vested interest in their bottom line.) Dr. Hitt had been using NAD+ in his drug and alcohol detox clinic since 1982, purchasing the NAD+ from South Africa, where a long-time employee had a relative.

After Hurricane Katrina, my husband and I opened a new clinic in Springfield, Louisiana, calling it Springfield Wellness Center. We have since treated more than 1,500 patients with intravenous BR+NAD™—and trained other physicians to do the same. The results have been phenomenal—or, as some people say, "too good to be true." We know differently.

NAD+ is a coenzyme found naturally in every cell in the human body. It's one of the four coenzymes of niacin, more commonly known as Vitamin B3, and is one of the chemicals responsible for cell metabolism—the transfer of energy from foods we eat into vital cell functions, including energy levels, cell repair, disease expression and suppression, aging, longevity, and more. NAD+ also helps restore brain functioning lost due to addiction, stress, depression, trauma, age, poor diet, chemotherapy, environmental toxins, and neurodegenerative diseases like Parkinson's and Alzheimer's. That's why we call our NAD+ formulation "Brain Restoration Plus"—it helps restore brain function—whether that means recovering from the effects of addiction to a single drug, or several.

Because NAD+ is an essential bionutrient, involved in so many bodily functions, when NAD+ levels are deficient, "almost all reactions in the body run down," as Dr. Abram Hoffer wrote in his foreword to the book: *NAD+ Therapy: Too Good to Be True?* [28] Hoffer was a Canadian psychiatrist with a Ph.D. in biochemistry who discovered a link between NAD+ deficiency and what had been diagnosed as schizophrenia, but which evaporated when NAD+ levels were restored. Throughout his career (1950-2009) Dr. Hoffer wrote more than 30 books on niacin/NAD+ treatment for a wide variety of illnesses and conditions. He believed that "NAD+ deficiency may be an unrecognized epidemic of cellular disease."

For example, from 1900-1945, some three million Americans were stricken with—and more than 100,000 died from—a disease called pellagra, which was rampant throughout the rural south. The result of niacin deficiency due to a diet that relied heavily

---

[28] Verwey, Theo, NAD+Therapy! Too Good to be True? 1989-2009; foreword by Abram Hoffer, MD, PhD.

upon corn, with little meat or other source of protein, pellagra manifested as the "four Ds"—dermatitis (painful skin lesions across the sun-exposed parts of the body), diarrhea, dementia, and death. Though the conventional wisdom attributed pellagra to exposure to a virus or toxin of some kind, U.S. Surgeon General Dr. Joseph Goldberger determined that the disease was, in fact, the result of niacin deficiency and righted itself when niacin supplements were given. He further found that a diet containing milk, eggs, meat, and other protein effectively prevented pellagra. Today the disease is found only in regions where the people consume a niacin-deficient diet. (Unfortunately, that can be many inner cities of the United States, where homeless people consume a mostly corn alcohol-based diet and many poor people subsist on corn-based breakfast cereal and milk.)

So, NAD+ is a coenzyme essential to the proper metabolic functioning of every cell in the body—and, for purposes of our discussion, the brain. The body can and does synthesize its own NAD+, and the body can also "salvage" or "recycle" NAD+ from "degraded" NAD+ products such as nicotinamide. However, when the body's NAD+ levels are overwhelmed and depleted, functioning is impaired, making a recovery from conditions like addiction extremely difficult. Unfortunately, oral NAD+ supplements are often insufficient, presumably because NAD+ breaks down during digestion. Another reason is probably that, in many NAD+ supplements, the dosage is too low. Moreover, the quality of the NAD+ supplement is critical. At Springfield Wellness Center, we have found that NAD+ potency, effectiveness, and shelf-life can vary widely by source, which is why we only stand by treatment results using NAD+ obtained from Archway Apothecary. However, when quality NAD+ is administered intravenously, the body—and its central processing unit, the brain—gets a reboot that can be transformative. Archway has independently tested various NAD+ products on the market and confirmed that they contain a lower purity than the 99.99% pure BR+NAD™ Archway produces.

Recent research shows that the body's NAD+ levels tend to decline with age, and that the deficiency accelerates with substance abuse. Also, some researchers believe that nearly 10% of the population is *born* with chronic NAD+ energy deficiency, or NED. This genetic component may support the known heredity of a spectrum of diseases, most notably, alcoholism.

NAD+ researchers believe that NAD+ energy deficiency induces fatigue and depression and increases the propensity to use drugs and alcohol to improve energy and mood. Oxidative stress associated with addiction and alcohol abuse unfortunately further decreases NAD+ levels. This self-medicating cycle is a common story reported by addicts. Unfortunately, it leads to even lower NAD+ levels.

Another function of NAD+ is to facilitate DNA repair. This is my favorite of NAD+'s multiple roles because it might be the explanation for what some patients call the "eraser effect," which occurs when a patient finds that all cravings and even thoughts of drinking or using are gone after a single treatment. They've said that they have to remind themselves that they used to drink or take drugs. Although these patients are the exception, not the rule, even some patients who slip or have relapses ultimately get the "eraser effect," provided they get enough BR+NAD™ over an extended period.

At Springfield Wellness Center, we use NAD+ as a primary treatment tool for clients seeking to break their chemical dependencies. When delivered intravenously, we've found that NAD+ very effectively—and relatively easily—helps to detox patients from a variety of substances—not only opiates but also alcohol, benzodiazepines, crystal meth, inhalants, bath salts, marijuana, and virtually every addictive compound, even GHB, Spice, and catnip.

What's unique about NAD+ is that, in addition to being

a non-addictive chemical that the body produces naturally, it dramatically reduces and, after a few days, eliminates the cravings that can make a recovery so difficult. NAD+ also removes the metabolites—the breakdown products—especially of alcohol detoxification, so it greatly reduces the length and intensity of withdrawal symptoms.

In the study[29] we presented at the November 2014 Society of Neuroscience meeting in Washington, D.C., my husband, Dr. Mestayer, our colleagues, and I documented that 60 adult patients (both male and female) with addictions primarily to opiates and alcohol reported that their cravings stopped or were significantly diminished. Their cravings fell from an average rating of five or six (on a 0 to 10 scale) on Day One to a rating of two by Day Five and an average of one or less by Day 10. The treatment in question consisted of our proprietary formulation of BR+NAD™, which is composed primarily of intravenous infusions of NAD+, along with oral amino acids and N-acetyl cysteine (NAC) for an average of 10 consecutive days. The treatment was administered from five to 10 hours daily at a dose range of 500 mg-1500 mg each day.

Because addiction's deleterious effects on NAD+ levels also affect the brain and central nervous system functioning, restoring brain function not only aids in addiction recovery, it also improves clarity, problem-solving ability, focus and concentration, energy levels, and overall sense of well-being. Some patients who have been in chronic pain also get a brain "reset" and *no longer need painkillers*. This is a huge bonus, which frequently escapes mention because patients are so impressed with their addiction recovery. However, the reduction of pain is likely a major factor in their success at staying clean: who needs a painkiller if you're not in pain? Clients describe feeling as if "life is worth living again." Their overall outlook is so

---

[29] Broom, Carson, Cook, Hotard, Mestayer, Norris, Simone & Stuller

positive—ebullient even—they can envision positive futures for themselves, which most have been unable to do for years.

In addition to significantly reduced cravings, BR+NAD™ recipients also report a dramatic reduction in withdrawal symptoms. These symptoms vary according to the chemical from which they are detoxing but typically include nausea, vomiting and muscle spasms for opiate withdrawal and tremors (DTs) for alcohol withdrawal, and deep depression for crystal meth withdrawal. We can generalize from our experience that withdrawal symptoms are reduced by 70 percent to 80 percent. This holds true no matter what patients have been addicted to—even methadone or Suboxone.

BR+NAD™ also appears to be effective in reducing or eliminating Post-Acute Withdrawal Syndrome (PAWS), which, along with cravings, is another reason for relapse. While PAWS can complicate opiate withdrawal for as long as a year or more under conventional addiction treatment protocols, BR+NAD™ appears to *eliminate* them initially and, if patients feel them coming back on, they can return for a "booster" re-treatment of a day or two, after which they become symptom-free again. Now that we have other delivery systems for BR+NAD™ (nasal spray, patches, cream, subcutaneous injections) these can be used in most cases instead of intravenous boosters. Each person's PAWS will respond differently based on the amount of oxidative stress the person experiences once they finish the BR+NAD™. Following the aftercare plan is essential in each case.

How does NAD+ work?

The exact reasons for NAD+'s effectiveness in addiction recovery are still being investigated. Although NAD+ has been medically utilized for drug rehab in South Africa since the 1970s, in Mexico since the 1980s, and has also been used during that time in the United States and Canada, treatment protocols—particularly for opiate addiction—have shifted primarily to methadone, and later Suboxone, as noted previously. In the interim, the patent for NAD+ expired—leaving pharmaceutical companies with little incentive to investigate its clinical properties and mechanism pathways. We are thrilled that a resurgence of interest in NAD+ research is currently under way—and that Springfield Wellness Center is in the center of it. I describe that research in greater detail in Chapter 12.

In the meantime, our own clinical experiences have led us to propose several theories regarding some of NAD+'s capabilities:

NAD+ improves alcohol metabolism because aiding metabolism is one of its primary functions overall. When metabolized, alcohol breaks down into a cascade of substances that also need to be metabolized—and NAD+ is also important in the breakdown of these byproducts. Although a healthy body has sufficient NAD+ levels to handle these metabolic tasks, chronic alcohol abuse drains the body's NAD+ reservoirs. By intravenously supplementing NAD+, we're able to give the body what it needs.

How NAD+ can reduce nausea and vomiting and muscle tremors is more difficult to say; however, we do know that NAD+, like vitamin C, is a tremendous antioxidant, so that may be part of the answer. Also, by giving the NAD+ intravenously, we bypass the stomach and go directly to the bloodstream, allowing NAD+ and its metabolites to be carried to the cells in the brain. Patients typically report feeling better, with increased mental clarity, within a few days, so long as the treatment regimen is followed.

For some people coming off of opiates, it is suspected that NAD+ probably helps to moderate and improve opiate receptor activity. Opiate receptors go into spasms when a patient attempts to quit the drug "cold turkey." However, NAD+ helps to alleviate these symptoms, although the exact mechanism has not been clinically demonstrated. Nevertheless, researchers *can* describe many ways in which NAD+ addresses oxidative stress and the genetic, epigenetic, and environmental factors that can result in addiction. More on that research is reported in Chapter 12.

At Springfield Wellness Center, our confidence in NAD+ effectiveness comes from treating more than 1,500 patients—and from the hundreds of additional patients who have been treated by our trained Fellows (see Chapter 13).

Our treatment differs from other addiction protocols because we begin by treating addiction as a brain disease. We understand that there are many emotional, psychological, and even spiritual factors that may lead to addiction—and also that, while addicted, patients often behave in ways that later require counseling to address—but we begin by helping the brain get back on track. We tell patients who enter our program that our intravenous treatment of BR+NAD™ will do three things:

1. It will detoxify them safely, with minimal withdrawal symptoms, and do so in two to four days depending on their addiction history.

2. Ninety-five percent of patients will have no cravings for their addictive substance by the end of treatment. Some will never have a craving again; others return periodically for a BR+NAD™ "booster," nasal spray, or the transdermal patch. (We have found that if patients return to a healthy environment, their prognosis for no subsequent cravings or relapse is good. If they return to a toxic environment, they may battle cravings again because their body has learned that strategy for coping with stress. My close relationship with one patient, James, is the reason I have been able to discover that in tough cases a person may need more than one BR+NAD™ treatment and a series of boosters over

time. It appears to me that, if indeed, BR+NAD™ has the ability to repair damaged DNA it must be based on dosage and intervals. How much a person receives and at what intervals they receive it shifts the balance to health in difficult cases.)

3. It will begin the process of restoring the brain to a level of clarity, function, and well-being that many haven't experienced since childhood.

What does this "Brain Restoration" effect look like? It is the visible transformation that makes my work so gratifying. I first notice a change in our patients' complexion: they get rosy cheeks, usually by the end of the first day of treatment or the start of the second day. Rosy cheeks are followed by "shiny eyes," by which I mean eyes that sparkle all the way across the room. Next come smiles, followed by happy chatter with other patients and staff. By days eight through 10, laughter dominates the room. Can you imagine a detox facility where the patients are giddy with laughter and euphoria?

In addition to offering BR+NAD™ as an addiction treatment, we also have found it effective for patients struggling with acute and chronic depression, anxiety, and post-traumatic stress disorder (PTSD). And, in the handful of cases we have tried, BR+NAD™ has even decreased symptoms of CTE (chronic traumatic encephalopathy—the disease described in the movie *Concussion*) and halted or reversed symptoms of Parkinson's and Alzheimer's.

Current research is beginning to unravel NAD+'s involvement in all of these various conditions. For example, research by Ling Shao and colleagues[30] at the University of

---

[30] Ling Shao,[1] Maureen V. Martin,[1] Stanley J. Watson,[2] Alan Schatzberg,[3] Huda Akil,[2] Richard M. Myers,[4] Edward G. Jones,[5] William E. Bunney,[1] and Marquis P. Vawter[1]. Mitochondrial Involvement in Psychiatric Disorders. <u>Ann Med. 2008; 40(4): 281–295.</u> https://www.ncbi.nlm.nih.gov/pmc/articles/PMC3098560/

California references a growing body of evidence implicating mitochondrial dysfunction in schizophrenia, bipolar disorder, and major depressive disorder. Investigations by our colleague and fellow psychiatrist, Dr. Elizabeth Stuller[31] confirm our results—that persons suffering from depression, anxiety, panic attacks, insomnia, irritability, anger, mania, and even psychosis respond well to intravenous BR+NAD™ treatment—enabling the brain to return to proper functioning.

By the time our patients come to us, they typically have tried many other treatment modalities. Most are reluctant to dare hope that our treatment can work where everything else has failed. It is such a joy for me to be able to assure them that if they give intravenous BR+NAD™ a try, it will not only enable them to break their addiction(s), it will do so with much less agony and discomfort than they've experienced before. Better still, when they're finished with our detox, they haven't exchanged one addiction for another.

Moreover, most of them are able to stay addiction-free after one treatment regimen. Others come back for a "booster" or even a full retreatment—and they do better the second time around than the first. They realize that even the euphoria of a drug-induced high is not as powerful as the feeling that their own health delivers.

Of course, patients also need to address the psychological, emotional, and even spiritual aspects of their addiction—not simply the physical reality of it. That means they must be committed to their aftercare—which not everyone is adequately motivated to do.

---

[31] Liz Stuller, MD, Brain Restoration Summit 2015 — NAD: The Future of Brain Health

*Hope is important because it can make the present
moment less difficult to bear. If we believe that tomorrow
will be better, we can bear a hardship today.*
—Thich Nhat Hanh

When our treatment doesn't work

Sadly, I know from experience that not *all* patients will receive what we hope for them. It would be great if everyone got the "eraser effect" like so many do, but they are the exception, not the rule. The majority of people we have treated do get very positive outcomes, but not all are that fortunate. Currently, we have a 90% success rate for eliminating cravings and restoring cognition in 10 little days of treatment. Most people find that hard to believe, but it doesn't matter. We see the results for ourselves and have seen the results consistently since 2001. There is no doubt in our minds that our treatment works; we just can't explain *how* to our satisfaction or to the satisfaction of other professionals in our field. We are keenly aware that IRB-approved clinical trials are necessary.

Here are some of the reasons why the outcomes sometimes fail to meet our expectations:

1. Some patients agree to treatment to please someone else. They are not yet invested in their own decision to let go of their addiction.
2. Some patients have had such bad experiences in other detox settings, or detox they have undertaken on their own, they will "use" during the treatment if withdrawal seems intolerable. We don't judge them or shame them if that happens; we just encourage them to trust us and stay the

course. We will get them to the other side of the withdrawal as soon as possible, and we will stay with them, we will not leave them. If we have to add a day or two of treatment to erase the damage done by using, we will.

3. Some patients are facing a life-changing event like a divorce, loss of a job, or a legal issue that heightens their stress while receiving the treatment. In those cases, they may get a good response, but the length of time it lasts can be shortened by the stress induced once they return home. Remember, NAD+ levels fluctuate for many reasons; stress is one of the major ones.

4. In cases where there is a dual diagnosis, like bipolar depression and addiction, once the addiction is addressed successfully, treatment of the mental health component needs to be supervised. In many situations, however, symptoms that present as a psychiatric disorder may be the result of substance abuse. What is exciting about BR+NAD™ treatment is that there may not *be* a psychiatric disorder once the substance is gone and the person is no longer using.

5. Sometimes the family, or spouse, or both, are exhausted by the time they reach out to us for help. The patient is exhausted, too. There is so much pent-up resentment on all sides that each person involved must be committed to repairing the emotional injuries the disease of addiction has caused the entire family unit. Otherwise, a positive short-term outcome may quickly evaporate once the patient returns home. Many people resist it, but the best thing for the family following our treatment is family therapy with a compassionate and skilled therapist.

6. Trusting the process is essential for the healing of addiction. Unlike other diseases, addiction is easily judged harshly through the lens of morality. Please remember not

to judge yourself or your family member harshly. Healing is a process; trust it and be patient with it.

Here are some clinical observations I've made over the years, which may be helpful for someone considering this treatment.

1. Everyone shows up with their own unique brain. No two brains are the same, and each must be individually treated based on individual medical history, current health status, and treatment response.
2. The age at which someone experiences chronic stress, trauma, or begins to use brain-altering chemicals is significant.
3. The level of motivation to feel better and the desire to make the necessary changes in lifestyle are important.
4. The age at which someone comes in for treatment affects the outcome. Adolescents are the high-risk group, for several reasons. First and foremost, the human brain is the last organ to fully develop and most scientists agree that it doesn't reach maturation, particularly for males, until somewhere between ages 22 and 28. Another reason is peer pressure. Being accepted by peers is very important for adolescents; in fact, it is more important than being accepted by parents (in case you haven't noticed)!
5. Patients who have had some success in their life before becoming addicted have a greater chance of maintaining sobriety or managing post-acute withdrawal symptoms after their treatment. Success in school, athletics, music, the arts, along with employment, professional achievements, business management, or other accomplishments will always be a foundation from which to return and succeed once again, when brain restoration has taken place.

6. If a person has a healthy, supportive family, they have an environment that can help maintain their sobriety. The supportive family unit is probably the strongest indicator of success, along with a strong spiritual, or faith-based, orientation to life. Practicing one's faith provides an anchor and a compass when the soul gets lost. I secretly believe that is why the people who come to us, find us.

7. The desire to be free from addiction must be strong. "You have to want it more than anything. You have to want it from your toes!" says precious Kim, who is five years without alcohol and who got the "eraser" effect.

8. There needs to be a willingness to embrace the challenges one faces when you return home. Those challenges include following your aftercare plan. In most cases, the plan includes the basics of wellness, which have kept some people free of addiction in the first place, such as regular exercise, healthy nutrition, keeping good company, smiling and laughing as often as you can, and stress management, including daily meditation and prayer. Inspirational material read right before falling asleep will resonate with you all night. Seeing a trustworthy therapist if you have not yet made peace with your anger and fear. Volunteering and being of service to other people or precious animals. Planting a tree in your honor and watching it grow with you. Gardening, fishing, playing tennis, golfing, singing, playing an instrument, painting, reading, and dancing as though no one is watching can all stimulate the reward center of your brain in healthy ways. Work on getting free and maintaining your freedom by being engaged in your life. Like Admiral William MacRaven says, "Make your bed!" Like Dr. Rick Rigsby says, "Find

your broom!" In other words, daily habits add up to discipline, and discipline adds up to success.

Our good fortune in finding Archway Apothecary

Since 2001 Springfield Wellness Center and its predecessor clinic have used four different intravenous NAD+ products to ease addiction detox. All but one of those products has been *lyophilized*, a process that diminishes the potency of the NAD+ due to the heat exposure it generates. The lyophilized products would range from 82% to 91% potency, and degrade over time. The one product we have found that is 99.99% pure and remains stable at that potency for 90-plus days is compounded by Archway Apothecary. Carl Camp and his team of pharmacists at Archway have figured out how to compound NAD+, a very fragile co-enzyme, without using the lyophilizing process. This benefits the patient because the purity improves the strength, maximizing efficacy, which dramatically shortens the uncomfortable withdrawal symptoms of detox.

To distinguish the Archway product from the other NAD+ products available, we named the Archway product BR+NAD™. I entered into a business relationship with Archway for the production of NAD+ products, bringing our treatment concepts and intellectual property to them in exchange for their expertise and compounding investment.

Archway Apothecary was formed in 2013 to serve the compounding needs of physicians and patients. Their state-of-the-art 6,000-square-foot facility was designed and constructed to meet the stringent USP 797 quality control requirements, with the ability to meet cGMP criteria should that become necessary in the future. Archway produces their compounds in accordance with the industry's strictest quality control standards. Contrast this with some of the NAD+ products imported from China, or elsewhere, with questionable, if any, quality controls. Archway Apothecary maintains an ISO Class 5 clean room, kept at an ideal 65 degrees F with 40% humidity, 365 days a year. In other words, it never deviates from this standard. Every six months the facility is inspected and its status confirmed by a third-party environmental control inspector in addition to periodic inspections by state regulatory authorities.

Archway's preparation of sterile, compounded BR+NAD™ for infusion is done completely within the requirements of USP 797 to ensure patients receive quality preparations that are free from contaminants and are consistent in intended identity, strength and potency. Each production lot of BR+NAD™ is tested by outside laboratories for sterility and potency before it is released to physicians. Results to date have shown NO batch failures!

Because we have tried NAD+ from other sources, we are convinced that the results we have achieved at Springfield Wellness Center are due to the quality, purity, and potency of the BR+NAD™ we use. In fact, that is why we certify other BR+NAD™ providers and insist that they source their BR+NAD™ *only* from Archway Apothecary. This is not because of some referral marketing scheme, but because we know from experience that BR+NAD™ delivers the results we have experienced. There's no telling what results others will experience using NAD+ sourced elsewhere, administered by improperly trained professionals.

We consider ourselves—and our patients—extremely fortunate to have crossed paths with Sam Camp, his sons Carl and Stephen, and the exceptional pharmacists, led by Ray Wilkes, at Archway Apothecary. They truly want to be of service to physicians and patients. They believe in our mission and have put their considerable skills to work on our behalf. Sometimes I feel like we are a tiny "think tank," continually working towards the well-being of our patients. When we meet, lots of laughter and an exchange of both promising and challenging ideas fills the room. We call each other "family," and I also believe the Camps are some of the "angels among us."

From science to compassion

Whatever the biochemical reasons for BR+NAD™'s effectiveness, one of the central tenets of our mission at Springfield Wellness Center is compassionate care. We understand that no one intends to become an addict. We understand how hard it can be to break the bonds of addiction, and how horrible it feels to be in the grip of something you cannot control. For this reason, addiction medicine is often referred to as "healing the hopeless." Our patients are exhausted. They are ill. They don't have access to their "right mind." They are spiritually, emotionally, physically, and financially fatigued.

But their situation is *not* hopeless. At Springfield Wellness Center, we know that their "right mind" can be returned to them. Carl C. Pfeiffer, MD, who also had a PhD in biochemistry and founded the Pfeiffer Medical Center, famously said that "For every drug that benefits a patient, there is a natural substance that can achieve the same effect." We know that to be true. The body's wisdom, properly supported through this common little coenzyme called NAD+, can liberate the most abject addict from despair. The dark night of the soul can be traversed. Even more exciting, the journey takes only 10 days, and we accompany our patients through every one of them.

Then, on treatment day 10 we have a joyful, silly graduation exercise, complete with goofy hats. We sing together *I Can See*

Clearly Now by Johnny Nash. Since ours is a secret society, I cannot reveal our induction passage or our secret handshake. I can tell you, though, that for every patient who leaves Springfield Wellness Center, rosy-cheeked and sparkly-eyed, we're reminded of the truth of our axiom, "It matters to this one!" from Loren Eiseley's story about the boy who kept throwing starfish back into the ocean despite the huge numbers of starfish still stranded on the beach. BR+NAD™ matters to each patient we reach.

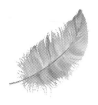

*The soldier above all prays for peace because it is the
soldier who bears the wounds and scars of war.*
—Gen. Douglas MacArthur

CHAPTER EIGHT

Today Is Veterans Day

Today is Veterans Day. It is a special day for me because we are a military family. I can say that proudly now, but I kept quiet during the Vietnam War. The violent demonstrations on campuses across the country intimidated me. My peers who were burning flags, bombing buildings, spitting in the faces of those who returned home from fighting, confused me. I was naïve. I was taught that our flag was a symbol of freedom and never to let it touch the ground. I was taught that I was not privileged because of who my father was. I was taught that respect, integrity, and honor were values to cherish. I couldn't quite justify in my adolescent mind why my peers didn't understand that it was our friends who were drafted that allowed them the freedom to demonstrate. I didn't feel like an "ugly American," which is what some of my peers claimed we were.

My father was a decorated veteran of WWII and Korea. He then spent over 28 years in the Army Corps of Engineers—ample time to get addicted to alcohol. His post-traumatic stress was held so tightly inside that at the age of 61 his heart exploded. He didn't talk about his war experiences until much later in his life when, while drinking at the kitchen counter, he would sometimes say, "I have to make peace with my Maker." If he left the room for a moment, I would try to water down his drinks. He was never abusive, but I didn't like the sadness in his eyes and the slurring of his speech. Sometimes I'd write him notes pleading with him to stop drinking.

I also call my father my first patient—because I was the daughter who listened to him at night during his drinking episodes. I hated to see the man I respected most change so dramatically because of a cocktail. I felt helpless—because he was far too proud to admit something was wrong. He told me once about a night in Korea when he made his rounds in the tents to make sure all his men were accounted for. As he walked down the center aisle, he noticed a soldier whose blanket had fallen off. He picked the blanket up and covered the young man—only to have the young soldier grab his hand tightly. My father held fast in return and stood there silently until the young man let go. No words were necessary. My father returned to his tent and began the arduous task of writing letters to the families of his fallen. He didn't say, but I imagine some bourbon helped him through the night.

Since those nights in the kitchen with my father, I've had the honor of treating many veterans struggling with alcohol, drug addiction, post-traumatic stress, and various combinations of all three.

One of them, Patrick, is a decorated Marine combat veteran who served two tours in Iraq and one in Afghanistan. When his father called to inquire about our treatment, he said his son was in trouble with heroin addiction. I explained what we do and how it differs from other detox treatments. "What is the cost?" his father asked. When I told him, he pleaded, "Don't you help veterans? He doesn't have that kind of money." My impulse to rescue surfaced immediately.

"How quickly can you get him here?" I asked.

Patrick came into my office in full-blown withdrawal. I took as much medical information as I could under the circumstances.

He had been prescribed 15 different medications at the VA, and when they took him off the pain medication, he turned to an alternative he could get "on the street"—heroin. He had refused to go back to the VA for counseling because the therapist "just typed into the computer and never made eye contact." (This is a complaint I've heard from many, not only of the VA but all hospitals, since the implementation of electronic charting.)

Patrick felt dismissed. He didn't feel like anyone cared. He was angry that no one apparently understood. Patrick had lost more than his buddies. He'd lost his wife and family, his job, his self-esteem. He had debilitating post-traumatic stress, which uneducated and insensitive civilians believe to be a weakness. He'd lost his physical and mental health, which had simply been medicated by the VA—in some cases exacerbating his condition.

I encouraged Patrick to trust that our treatment would work if he would commit to 10 days of intravenous BR+NAD™. Although I could not truly understand what he was going through, I told him that I was an army brat and had indirectly experienced some of what he must be feeling. And that, from our experience treating other veterans, I was certain he would be victorious in his fight against his addiction. But when I said we couldn't begin treatment until the next morning, Patrick abruptly stood up and said "Let's go. They can't help me."

I assured Patrick that we *could* help him and we would start first thing the next morning. I prayed that night for his return, knowing fully well that his withdrawals that night would be excruciating.

Patrick did show up, and we got him started right away. He was so sick he had to stay on the daybed, but he was a Marine and fought his way through. Because he had a sensitive gut, we had to slow the delivery of the BR+NAD™, taking us two days to get one day's worth of serum into his system. Not wanting him to give up, I asked him to stay with us overnight.

On the morning of the third day, Patrick got out of the bed

and, walking toward us, said, "Last night was the first time in seven years I didn't have a nightmare!" That was the beginning of a BR+NAD™ miracle. I had no idea that BR+NAD™ (on its own, without psychotherapy) could begin to heal post-traumatic stress. We did engage in several months of psychotherapy after that first BR+NAD™ treatment, which helped to resolve some of the trauma of combat, but the additional boosters supporting our psychotherapy fueled our success. Patrick kept returning to us for a booster treatment every six to eight weeks initially, until now he receives a booster annually, or whenever he feels his anxiety ratcheting up. Today, Patrick has been drug-free for more than eight years and is off all of the medications the VA prescribed for him. He has received the "eraser effect." His experience has taught us that, for some addiction patients, or those who also deal with trauma or extreme pain, the eraser effect comes over time, following repeated treatment. That is good news.

The other night I received a text from Patrick, who wrote, "I just wanted to thank you for everything. I would not trade the life you and Doc gave me back for anything." This morning, Veterans Day, I thanked him for his service.

Douglas is another veteran we treated for post-traumatic stress and addiction. Douglas served nine years in the army, including two deployments in Iraq and one in Afghanistan. He had severe post-traumatic stress when he returned to the States. He had started using drugs at the age of 14, and his history included cocaine, heroin, speed, Suboxone, pain pills—anything and everything. He was a "high-functioning addict" until the day he drove his car through a McDonald's and was sent to a 30-day detox treatment program in Texas.

Douglas had detoxed previously on 19 separate occasions before coming to us. He was facing detox from Suboxone, which he calls, "10 times worse than heroin to quit." But after 10 days of intravenous BR+NAD™ therapy, he was clean. He had "one bad day," he says, but it was nowhere near the bad days he'd had on previous withdrawal attempts.

Douglas had been scheduled to complete a 90-day addiction treatment program at a VA hospital when he left us, but when he reported as scheduled, he had no trace of drugs in his bloodstream. The staff accused him of lying about his addiction. He has now been clean and free of cravings for more than three years and feels so good he stopped counting his days of sobriety after Day 80. His hypervigilance and post-traumatic stress symptoms are gone, as well. His life has so changed that he has returned to school to get a degree in psychology so that he can better understand addiction and help people like himself. Our former patient Patrick ran into him selling cars to help pay his way through school! They shared their joy at beating their common demons.

So many vets I've treated wanted to return to active duty because that is where they'd felt most alive, most respected, and most appreciated. They felt a duty to "have the backs" of the buddies they'd left behind. They are talented and disciplined, but now can't hold down a job—because when the flashbacks come crashing in, and they see dead buddies coming through the walls of their bedroom, they have nowhere to turn for help without being labeled crazy. So, they are afraid to sleep. Sleep-deprived and under the influence of mind-altering substances, they are short-tempered, unable to concentrate, and their hypervigilance stays with them in restaurants, at ballgames, and even while driving their car. I've known vets to sleep under the bed with their backs to the wall. Many hide their flashbacks from their family and friends so their loved ones won't be afraid of them. Thousands self-medicate with the wrong stuff…alcohol, opiates, benzos, cocaine, methamphetamines, and anything else they can get their hands on to numb the pain. That, of course, makes for a mess of their relationships—not only relationships with spouses and family members, but also with themselves. They don't recognize or want to claim the person they feel they have become. That is why we nurture them without judgment or criticism. We don't tell them, as some do, that if "their lips are moving they must be lying." Rather, we let them know that most people lie because they are afraid. We know that they sincerely, desperately want to get well, but they are afraid they can't. We also know that in 10 short days the real human being—Keith, Joe, Sally, or Mary—will return. It is a gift to behold for those of us who are privileged to lead them through their despair to their redemption.

To get off opiates for pain, or benzos for anxiety or depression, involves a high degree of medical management and supervision. Just sending someone home with a daily regimen of pills isn't going to do what is needed. People struggling with pain, depression, anxiety, or all three, need a therapeutic bond with a compassionate professional. Veterans do, in particular, but all those who suffer from addiction and post-traumatic stress require a relationship based on trust to support them through the times of self-doubt and panic.

We have learned that there is no substitute for compassion in the practice of mental health and addiction treatment. To listen respectfully to the patient's message opens the corridor to all the rooms in which secrets are kept. To be invited into one or more of these rooms is a sacred gift and should be honored as such. Some rooms are easier to enter than others. Some rooms are locked, but authentic compassion may help the patient find the key and the willingness to venture in, with us by their side. *When their pain is greater than their fear*, they will act differently and begin to renovate their lives. Truth and integrity are the hallmarks of treatment success. No guilt, no shame, no judgment are essential to achieving it.

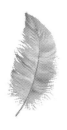

The voyage of discovery is not in seeking new
landscapes but in having new eyes.
—Marcel Proust

CHAPTER NINE

The Qi Runs Through It

Qi, or *chi*, or *ch'i*, is a Chinese term for the spiritual energy, or life force, running through all things. *Feng shui* is the art of designing physical spaces to harmonize with the *qi* in their environment; to optimize, or at the very least not block, the *qi*. I was delighted to learn that the Chinese characters for *feng shui* mean "wind-water" because wind and water are a very important part of what makes Springfield Wellness Center such a special, healing place. The *qi* runs through it.

Springfield Wellness Center is located in a small town in Louisiana—a town marked by one traffic light, one post office, one drug store, and one grocery store. It is perhaps a surprising, unassuming place for miracles or magic to happen. Why would someone from Manhattan, Boston, Palm Beach, Los Angeles, Brasilia, London, or Sydney come all the way to Springfield, Louisiana? Some come because they are wearied from the fight against the fear, nightmares, and shame of addiction, or the chronic physical pain that robs them of their sleep, their jobs, their relationships. A few come because they are curious to see what the heck we are doing in the Louisiana swamp. Like many explorers, they want to see for themselves: is the world flat or not?

My husband often jokes that what we are doing at Springfield

Wellness is a result of Attention Deficit Disorder (ADD)—mine. Who, but someone with ADD, would bypass the rehab center located right across the street and go all the way to Tijuana, Mexico, to seek out help for her daughter, as I did?

He is referring to a theory about ADD and ADHD (Attention Deficit Hyperactivity Disorder) by Thom Hartmann. In his book, *Attention Deficit Disorder: A Different Perception*, Hartmann proposed that those with ADD had "hunter brains," always on the move, alert to every sound in the environment, willing to take risks; while those without the "disorder" have "farmer brains," patient, methodical, and able to focus on a task over long periods of time.

My retort to my husband, and to any patient who shares this condition and has not yet realized it is an asset, is that ADD confers membership in a very special club. Hundreds of famous people are members of the ADD club, and their contributions to the world are legendary. I often ask, "Do you know who our first club president was?" They don't, so I tell them: "Christopher Columbus! Who but an ADDer could persuade the Queen of Spain to finance his trip off the edge of the earth with three ships, fully manned, fully supplied, to see whether the world is flat and if not, bring home the gold and other shiny stuff?" That's what we ADDers do; explore the world in different ways. We take risks; we want to know why; we like to keep moving, we learn—only differently!

That is why I took my daughter to Mexico once I discovered that she had begun to experiment with drugs and alcohol. I took her to Mexico because I had heard about a doctor there who was doing detoxification treatment for drug and alcohol abuse which he called Neurotransmission Restoration (NTR). That was in 1998, and although our trip was not financed by any King or Queen curious about the shape of the planet or looking for gold or other riches, I did discover what my husband called the Treasure of the Sierra Madre—elusive, but we found it. At the outset, that exploratory journey to Mexico was intended to help and protect my daughter. As fate would have it, that journey brought me from NTR to BR+NAD™ and Springfield, Louisiana.

Springfield Wellness Clinic is housed in a modest Acadian "Dog Trot" cottage, situated on a 500-acre estate owned by my dear friend Debra Neill Baker, who is the president and chairman of the Neill Corporation. She has always believed in me and has supported our efforts to provide effective mental health treatment, as well as develop and expand our services and knowledge of the use of BR+NAD™. Debra and I go back a long way, but ours is a friendship outside of space and time. Once I remarried, we didn't see each other for years, but after Hurricane Katrina, she offered the "Dog Trot" to us since we lost our clinic to the storm. I had been sharing space in another clinic when Debra and I reconnected and made plans to meet for lunch. While she waited for me in the clinic waiting room, the patient I had just seen for anxiety appeared at the door of the waiting room and said in a dreamy voice, "I love coming here." Debra told me as we left for lunch, "I want what she got!"

Shortly after that we moved into the Dog Trot and never left!

I almost feel superstitious about the place. I'm afraid to move to a larger location, even though the staff keeps saying we need a bigger boat. The Dog Trot is a name given to a rustic architectural design of Cajun origin, consisting of a large open center hall and four separate rooms opening off of it, two on either side. In earlier times, the hall was open, so on hot summer days, the dogs could lie in the hall to cool off as the wind blew through. "Cajun A/C," you might imagine. The old house was moved to Debra's property 25 years before and was renovated to its present condition, with indoor plumbing, central air and heat, a well-equipped kitchen with a Wolf range, and beautifully landscaped grounds. It is serene. It is peaceful. It is comfortable. John Melhourn, one of our addiction counselors, calls it "The Nest."

I playfully say the *qi* runs through the place because a *feng shui*-minded architect designed two ponds to be built on either side of the house. The north and south entrances of the center hall open onto the grounds surrounding both ponds. In the philosophy of *feng shui*, it is said, *"Qi* rides the winds and scatters, but is retained when encountering water." How does that affect the Dog Trot? The *qi* rides the wind blowing through the hall but encounters the ponds, which then keep the *qi* flowing in a circular motion. Why is that important? According to this Chinese system of thought, *qi* is the force that binds nature and humans together. With proper architectural considerations, the *qi* can bring health, prosperity, and happiness.

Hundreds of individual testimonies confirm the healing energy of Springfield Wellness Center. This invisible force called *qi, shakti*, or by some, *Holy Spirit*, may be the energy behind the miracles we witness almost daily.

Unmistakable signs: providence or coincidence?

One such example was TJ, a young man of 22, who was already a full-blown alcoholic. He had completed two residential treatment programs and was now in the diversion program with the court system. He simply could not stop drinking. No treatment or recovery program had worked, and he felt hopeless and trapped. Springfield Wellness Center is often a person's last resort. This was true for TJ. His life seemed impossible, given the circumstances he had to face and the loss of his dreams. His high school sweetheart had given birth to his baby girl, but they had not married. Rather, they lived separately with their parents. Instead of going to college, TJ worked in his father's business to pay for his expenses and those of his little girl. The only time his eyes would shine was when he talked about his daughter.

TJ and I connected in a very significant way, quickly forming a strong therapeutic alliance. TJ was an intellectual who read voraciously instead of watching movies or playing games on his iPad like some of the other patients.

Each day of treatment I monitor the rate of the intravenous infusion, which affects the level of comfort or discomfort a patient feels. I make sure they are as comfortable as possible and will cover them with a blanket, gently tuck them in, or wiggle a toe and give them words of encouragement. Often it is then that they begin to talk, ask questions, and assess whether I am to be trusted. When they are feeling better, I will often joke and ask if they are ready to come to the "principal's office," which is code for counseling. Their body language tells me if they are willing. If not, I wait for another opportunity and encourage them to meet with me when they feel safe.

In one such encounter, TJ asked me why I had decided to study psychology. He indicated that he had always been interested in psychology and wondered if he could pursue such a dream. I was in a playful mood, so I told him, "I look for the signs and follow the signs." His face told me he didn't understand, so I told him my story about going off to college and feeling full of fear, self-doubt, and depression as I started my journey toward my degree. I told him about praying for a sign that I was doing what I was supposed to do when behold, I saw my name carved into the windowsill of my dormitory room. TJ had a difficult time believing me. I assured him that it was indeed a true story that had given me the encouragement to face some of my fears and persevere.

My advice to TJ was to keep his eyes open for the magic in his life. To use not only his physical eyes but also the eyes of his soul, which can see things the physical eyes often miss. Signs are everywhere once you train yourself to start looking for them.

One day when TJ was ready to come "to the principal's office," we discussed his aftercare plan, which included attending the Celebrate Recovery meetings at his church. He was to finish his treatment the next day when I realized that I had been remiss in never asking him what he considered his primary "trigger." When fighting this disease, it is best to avoid people, places, and things that can generate cravings. To my dismay, he said his trigger was, "My job." He described how he would drink himself to sleep each night, wake up with a hangover, stop at a gas station to buy a pint of vodka, which he would consume after throwing up in the men's room once he got to work. That would get him through the day until he could go home and start this routine again. This had been his life for years.

My mind raced with thoughts of what I could do to help him since he was due to go to work the next day. Without sounding any alarms, I did say that we had a challenge to face because we had to do something to protect him at his job.

I asked him to close his eyes and pretend with me for just a little while. He sat quietly and followed my instructions of breathing diaphragmatically. We took several deep breaths before I asked him to see if he could imagine himself getting into his car to go to work. I asked him if he could imagine himself stopping at the gas station to get the pint of vodka. He said he could in both cases. I asked him if he could imagine arriving at his job and getting out of his car. He said he could, so I asked him to describe what he was wearing. He told me and then imagined himself walking into the building. At this point, I asked him to imagine walking toward the men's room, but this time the door of the men's room would be different. This time he would see a sign; a bright red circle with a line through it that means STOP/NO.

To his surprise and mine, he began to cry and suddenly opened his eyes repeating, "I don't cry! I don't cry!" By that time my eyes were teary too, so I told him that crying is a good thing.

It is a necessary part of our human experience; a safety valve that keeps us healthy. Certainly, at Springfield, we cry freely because we are here to be healthy. I assured him that crying had nothing to do with whether or not a person was strong. In fact, crying deeply with someone else is an ultimate compliment. When we share at that level of intimacy, we demonstrate trust and claim the strength of self. It is one of the most sacred of shared human experiences. To change his focus from embarrassment and shame, I told him about some research I'd read years ago about the chemical makeup of tears. I speculated that it was a woman who conducted the study because what man would study tears? In our culture, men are allowed to be half a human being. They are permitted to be happy, or angry, but they cannot show fear or sadness.

At any rate, the researcher who analyzed tears discovered that "onion-induced" tears were basically a saline solution. But emotional tears contain endorphins—which are the body's painkillers—along with dopamine and serotonin, two other feel-good chemicals—which explains why crying is so therapeutic. The definition of a healthy human being is that they have access to all the human emotions and can appropriately express them. So, every healthy person needs to be able to cry.

To lighten things up, we closed the session with a "pinky promise" that he would call me after work the next day. He did. I asked him if he'd had any cravings, which he answered by asking whether "thoughts" were considered cravings. I told him thoughts could stimulate physical responses, which could ultimately lead to physical cravings. He said, if that was the case, then yes, because he'd had thoughts about drinking most of the day. I asked him if he had used his nasal spray, a BR+NAD™ product made by Archway Apothecary, which is an aftercare bridge to manage cravings or anxiety or any other post-acute withdrawal symptom. He had not yet picked up the prescription, so I told him to get it before going to work the next day and to let me know if he had any cravings by the end of the day. The next afternoon I received the following text:

This morning I went to Archway to pick up my nasal spray before going to work. I had one thought today, so I used the spray an extra time, and the thoughts stopped within five minutes, which is a miracle for me! Oh, and by the way, I saw a sign today. Every day for the last three years I have seen a billboard on my way to work that says "Taaka Vodka, just add people." Today that billboard was different. Today it said, "Celebrate Recovery"!

Now THAT is a sign.

Jason's story

It was late afternoon when Jason came in for his assessment. An attractive young man with worry on his face, even though he smiled, he was eager to tell me why he was there, but first he wanted to know more about our treatment. As I began to explain what we do and how it might help him, he stopped to ask if this really was a brain reboot or a brain restoration treatment like he saw on the internet. I explained that our treatment does three things: detoxes patients safely with minimal withdrawals; blocks cravings; and yes, restores brain function, which we call "the brain restoration" piece.

He looked at me intently as he began to tell me his story. When he was 14 years old he began smoking marijuana. He was home alone and frightened that his parents would return and catch him. The TV was on and a news story about a new addiction detox treatment in Mexico that could restore the brain was reported. He described listening to the report and telling himself that if he ever got into trouble with drugs he could always go and get the treatment described on the evening news.

I listened but was puzzled as he described that he was now 34 and definitely in trouble with drugs. His addictions were causing problems with his family, especially his father with whom he shared a business. Also, the distance it was causing in his marital relationship was scary because he loved his wife more than anything else in his life. He needed help, so he searched "brain reboot" on the web and Springfield Wellness came up.

We looked at each other simultaneously with a bit of astonishment. Could it really be? Could this really be the program mentioned on television twenty years before? Was I the lady who was interviewed?

The answers were yes, and yes, and yes! We laughed out loud and signed him up for treatment. As I write this, Jason is now more than five-years drug free!

So, let me ask you: Is that a coincidence, or the *qi, shakti,* or Holy Spirit running through our work here, at Springfield Wellness Center?

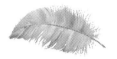

"And now here is my secret, a very simple secret: It is only with the heart that one can see rightly; what is essential is invisible to the eye."
—Antoine de Saint-Exupéry

Another example of the healing q*i* running through Springfield was that of a loving father who brought his adult son in for treatment. His son was hurting, frightened and angry, his brain ravaged by drug abuse. Each day, his father would have to force him to get up and come for treatment, which the young man would sometimes physically resist. Still, the father never left his side. The two kept with the treatment plan, while we nurtured, and nurtured, and nurtured, promising them from experience that they would soon be on the other side of the tunnel of despair. In this case, Day Five was the miracle day. The father came in with his son, who was beginning to feel better. As his son walked toward the nurses' station to receive his treatment, his father took me aside and began to tell me a story with tears in his eyes. He said that when his son was a toddler and would skin his knee, he would run to his father for comfort. When his father held him, the boy would put his head on his shoulder and rub his father's ear very softly to soothe himself. This particular morning there had been no physical altercation, no vulgar language, at the prospect of coming for treatment. Because his son was weakened by his disease, his father had bent down to help him get out of bed. When he did so, his son sat up and put his head on his father's shoulder and then began to rub his father's ear! Father and son reconnected in a very deep way that some fathers and sons never get to experience. This father took it as a sign that his son was reconnecting with his true self. I agreed.

It is worth mentioning that, though rare, in some cases a treatment regimen may be interrupted by unforeseen circumstances. If a patient completes 10 consecutive days of treatment and follows the individually designed protocol, most alcohol patients finish detoxing and report no cravings by day two or three. Opiate patients finish detoxing and report no cravings by day four or five, depending on their use history. Other addictions can fall within those parameters, but occasionally the type of substances used and the length of time using the substances can extend the treatment beyond the typical 10 days.

When we have to extend treatment in individual cases, we continue in the same fashion until we see the results we are looking for: no withdrawal symptoms, no cravings, improved mood, decreased anxiety, rosy cheeks, and sparkling eyes. In some cases, we can take a four-day recess and resume treatment with the next rotation. We currently work on a schedule of two 10-day rotations a month with a four-day recess between each rotation.

Our experience has shown us that the body's NAD+ levels are always fluctuating. I have noticed that the need for boosters is deferred as a person receives more BR+NAD™ over time. It appears that the key to success lies in the dosage and intervals of receiving the BR+NAD™. In some cases, I wonder if the answer is due, in part, to the repair of damaged DNA.

Explorers in all fields often discover things by accident. Major discoveries have been made just by watching bad weather! Observation is essential. At Springfield Wellness Center, we have used the power of observation to develop our addiction detox treatment protocols (BR+NAD™), since 2001. We started with addiction detox treatment only and adjusted and individualized our protocols based on our observations and patient feedback. Our protocols are fluid. We change them as we learn more about how the brain responds. We are open to collaboration in our search to find the most effective treatment for the disease of addiction—as well as other brain "diseases," including chronic traumatic encephalopathy (CTE), traumatic brain injury (TBI), and neurodegenerative diseases like Alzheimer's and Parkinson's. From our observations—and from current research that is being done—BR+NAD™ is a critical piece of the puzzle. We intend to discover as much as we can about NAD+'s implications for brain restoration and health through our recently established research foundation, NAD+ Research, Inc. (See Chapter 12.)

The "Watch Man"

Earlier I told you about a patient we came to call "the Watch Man" because of his poignant plea to accept his watch for payment, so desperate was he to get treatment for his addiction to pain meds.

The Watch Man's treatment was successful. Although he continued to see me for counseling for about a year afterward, I did lose contact eventually. I didn't know how successful his treatment had been until seven years later when I got a late-night phone call from a desperate wife of an alcoholic. When I lose contact with a patient, the voice in my head generally flip-flops between "They are okay; they've just resumed their lives," to "They have relapsed and are too embarrassed to call for a booster." I didn't know how the Watch Man was doing until that call seven years later.

The woman on the phone, Mrs. Smith, and her husband were both highly educated, retired seniors. Both had had successful careers with very little time for much other than their work. With retirement, though, Mrs. Smith became aware that her husband was drinking too much and was hiding the fact. In fact, he was even lying about it. In desperation, Mrs. Smith searched the phone book for the number of Alcoholic Anonymous. Unbeknownst to Mrs. Smith, she had misdialed the number. She told the person who answered that she was calling AA to get help for her husband. The voice on the other end told her she had dialed the wrong number but that he would advise her to call Springfield Wellness Center and ask for Paula

Norris. He was certain she would be helped. When she asked for his name, he simply said, "Tell her Bruce sent you."

The Alzheimer sister

What partially fueled the development of our research foundation (see Chapter 12) were the accidental discoveries we stumbled upon. For example, we had no idea that intravenous BR+NAD™ would help in neurodegenerative diseases associated with aging. One day a family of five came in to see if our treatment might help the one who was diagnosed with Alzheimer's disease. I met with them and explained we only treated people who are addicted to substances or had issues with stress, anxiety, or depression.

"But doesn't your treatment restore the brain?" they asked. I emphasized that our experience was limited to restoring the brain due to damage that was done by substances, not to any neurodegenerative disorders. They were insistent that they wanted to try anyway because they did not trust traditional medicine and wanted to take the chance that BR+NAD™ might just be helpful. The family almost begged me to at least give it a try once they knew that BR+NAD™ certainly would not hurt. They loved their sister very much and didn't want to see her suffer.

I left the room to discuss the situation with my husband, Dr. Mestayer, only to have him tell me sternly, "We don't treat Alzheimer's."

"Then *you* go in and tell them No," I said.

We walked back into the room together, and the family sitting there with expressions of prayerful anticipation began again to make a case for their sister to receive the treatment. My husband is a "softy" too, so instead of saying no, we began to make plans to give the treatment, with the clear understanding that we had no idea if it would help. We had not administered BR+NAD™ for this purpose before and would have to develop a protocol as we progressed. Because we knew it could not hurt her at our protocol dosages, we took the chance to see if it would help.

When we began, the sister with Alzheimer's was oriented only to herself. She got lost in the bathroom. She needed help with all self-care needs. She had a "flat affect" (a blank expression) and a distant stare. Each day of treatment produced an improvement over the previous one until she was "present" and smiling and talking to all of us. Her gait was also improved. Six days into treatment she was nearly fully cognizant of those around her. We asked that they return in three weeks for a follow-up appointment. They did return—and this time their sister came walking into the clinic with confidence and said to me, "Paula, you know the people who take care of me, my home health aides? They get on my nerves. Sometimes I pretend I don't know what they are saying just to get them to leave me alone."

It was a dramatic meeting. We were astonished at the remarkable difference in her condition. After the family left, my husband turned to me and said, "So now what are we going to do?" I smiled broadly saying, "I guess we will continue to help the people who show up and do what we can to be of service."

Friends don't let friends get Alzheimer's

This case paved the way for others with neurodegeneration to try the treatment. Billy, one of my dearest friends, was diagnosed with Alzheimer's and kept it a secret from me. When I found out, I threatened him with a black Suburban ride with a black hood over his head if he didn't come to see me. He agreed only if his neurologist would give him the okay. I told him his doctor wouldn't know what he was talking about, but suggested that he have his doctor call Dr. Mestayer, who would be able to answer any questions he might have. Billy's treatment plan included six days of intravenous BR+NAD™ infusions, followed by a one-day booster infusion each month for maintenance. We also gave him liposomal curcumin (the "active ingredient" in turmeric) and resveratrol and other supplements.

When Billy began treatment, his mental status exam score was 20, out of a possible score of 30. His kind and gentle personality was present, but noticeably absent were the twinkle in his eyes and the warm smile he typically wore. Instead, his expression had a dullness I had never seen.

A few months after his treatment, Billy had to take another mental status exam. He was worried about how well he would do because it was a longer, two-hour exam—not like the first one when he'd scored 20. He wasn't sure the two scores would be comparable. However, to his—and his neurologist's—surprise, his score was 24! His doctor called to give us the good news. This was not the normal progression for an Alzheimer's patient, who typically will lose two points each year following the diagnosis. But Billy's score had gone in the other direction—significantly! At his most recent exam—in January 2018—Billy's score was 29 out of 30! In fact, he no longer fits the profile of a person with Alzheimer's.

My husband had known Billy was improving because they are fishing buddies. For the same reason, my husband had been one of the first to know that something was amiss with Billy because he would get lost in the marsh and have to text my husband for help finding his way back to the dock. Billy no longer gets lost; he also remembers all the "secret" fishing holes. We also get text messages from mutual friends who thank us for "bringing Billy back" to them. Billy comes in once a month for a half-day booster, and all seems stabilized. His daughter, whom I first met vis-à-vis an ultrasound, is getting married soon. She is a truly beautiful young woman I've watched grow up. My heart smiles knowing that her mother, Suzy and I will get to watch her father walk her down the aisle with full cognition.

It is thanks to the groundbreaking work of Drs. Ross Grant, Jade Berg, and Nady Braidy of Australia (see Chapter 12) that Billy will be present at his daughter's wedding and remember giving her hand to her future husband. These insightful researchers, particularly Dr. Berg, showed that NAD+ levels in the brain decline with age and the cumulative effect of oxidative damage—from diet, environmental toxins, chronic stress, alcohol, drug, and pharmaceutical use, illness, and more. The level of oxygen necessary for the brain to maintain robust neurochemical activity is enormous. According to Dr. Grant, more than 100,000 chemical reactions happen every second. What is needed to sustain that demand? A constant supply of NAD+.

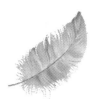

*Many of life's failures are people who did not realize
how close they were to success when they gave up.*
—Thomas A. Edison

CHAPTER TEN

Accidental Discoveries

Years ago, when we started using BR+NAD™, it was only in our detox treatment for addiction. Yet our frame of reference, mental health, has been instrumental in helping us develop our protocols for administering the treatment. Without our years of mental health practice, we would have been at a great disadvantage in understanding and addressing the inherent issues that accompany addiction detox and treatment: the withdrawal symptoms, the underlining conditions such as ADHD, anxiety, depression, bipolar disorder, psychosis, personality disorders, post-traumatic stress, or grief and bereavement, just to name a few. Addiction treatment would be simple if the only thing needing to be addressed was a substance dependency; but of course, the substance is only the tip of the iceberg.

If you are a professional considering using intravenous NAD+ without recognizing the mental health aspects of treatment, you may naively find yourself in a quandary. There is so much more to offering this treatment than meets the eye. Just ask Dr. Louis Cataldie, an addiction specialist, for whom I have immense respect, who wrote the book, *10,000 Addicts Later.* His book is a must-read for anyone considering doing this work, even if they have years of experience in administering intravenous infusion therapies of other kinds (such as vitamin C, Myer's Cocktails, hangover remedies, etc.)

That is the reason we train and certify our BR+NAD™ Fellows (and require that they *only* administer 99.99% pure BR+NAD™ compounded by Archway). For better or worse, clinics offering NAD+ infusions have proliferated in recent years. When Springfield Wellness Center held its first Brain Restoration Summit, in October 2015, there were only four websites advertising NAD+ addiction treatment. Two years later, there are dozens of pages of sites touting "NAD+"—including some who use the acronym to mean only "Natural Addiction Detox."

On the other hand, a growing number of clinics are staffed by providers we endorse, while still others are working towards their Fellowship status in our training certification program. (See Chapter 13) We are thrilled to train and qualify as many new Fellows as possible because we know there are millions of suffering people who could benefit. However, as much as we want to increase the number of qualified clinicians, we also want to prevent the proliferation of unqualified providers—because nothing will give NAD+ a bad name faster than uninformed or misguided people administering "NAD" in name only and failing to get good results.

We encourage anyone who would like to become a trained and certified BR+NAD™ provider to contact us. (See Chapter 13.)

NAD+ and the treatment of other conditions

We had no idea how valuable BR+NAD™ could be to neurodegenerative disease patients until by chance we were given opportunities to test it. We have always known that NAD+ is important to the brain and that the amounts we give are safe, so when patients started asking us to treat their conditions, we felt compelled to try. To our surprise, we were once again pioneering a new treatment option.

Two more Alzheimer's stories

Frankie's story is a haunting one for me. Frankie was my "brother from a different father and mother." We'd met at the age of 15 during our sophomore year of high school. He was a Navy brat. We discovered that our dads had been stationed in Hawaii at the same time, which meant we were both on the island of Oahu during elementary school, but we did not meet then. We developed a lifelong friendship. He was my big brother who seemed to have a radar alerting him to my ups and downs of growing up. We went different ways for college, but he was often there in my times of need. One of my regrets is missing his wedding to Olympia, the perfect mate for the rest of his life. I would always see him at high school reunions, and we would twist "like we did last summer" to Chubby Checker. (Funny how music has changed!)

I invited Frank and Olympia to my husband's 60th birthday party. It was then that I realized something had gone awry. In the bustle of entertaining a house full of guests, I realized that Frank could not speak properly. His words were not discernable. Olympia told me that he had been diagnosed with Alzheimer's disease. This was long before we knew how important NAD+ is for neurodegenerative diseases.

Nevertheless, I suggested he take our treatment, but because he did not have an addiction and he was taking medication for his condition, we didn't push him or insist that he try. The last time I saw him was at my mother's house, where we had spent a lifetime of camaraderie. I wasn't sure he would recognize me based on Olympia's warning, but he did and started crying. We embraced each other and cried until we took a seat on the sofa, where we sat without any space between us and just smiled at each other, without saying anything. Words were not necessary.

I think Frank's neurodegenerative disease was partly due to rugby; a rough contact sport played without protective gear. Frank played the game internationally and coached the sport for a time at the University of West Florida. How I wish now that we had treated him with BR+NAD™ when we might have had a chance to make a difference.

Another Alzheimer's treatment story has a happier ending. When I met Celeste, she was sitting at a table by herself. She was elderly and fidgeting with her fingers as she glanced about the room wide-eyed with anxiety. It was the 50th wedding anniversary of a couple who were celebrating in a large room full of family and friends. Celeste was supposed to know those in attendance but she didn't recognize anyone. For some reason, I went over to introduce myself and see if I could help her in some way. Her daughter, who was standing nearby, introduced herself and Celeste and explained that Celeste had a 10-year history of dementia labeled Korsakoffs-Alzheimer's. We talked a bit about how I might be able to help, so I left my name and phone number on a napkin in case they wanted to consider our treatment for neurodegenerative diseases. A couple of weeks later, Celeste and her daughter walked into the clinic with the hope that maybe, just maybe, our treatment might help.

Upon her arrival, Celeste was in the same shape as she was at the party. She knew her own name but did not know her daughter, or the names of other family members and friends who visited her on her first three days of treatment. However, over the next three days, Celeste's blank stare began to slowly slip away. In its place rose a relaxed expression, bright eyes, and a smile. When she walked around the clinic, her personality was playful and she was flirtatious with the doctors and male nurses. She sat in one of the lounge chairs in the treatment room across from another patient, named Bubby. By day five most patients are feeling so much better that their laughter, giggles, and chatter contribute to a relaxed and safe environment where people interact with very little inhibition. It was day four when Celeste called for her daughter by name, Alecia. It had been two long years since Alecia had heard her mother say her name and actually recognize her. She was consumed by joy.

It was day five when Bubby came up to me in complete astonishment at the progress he had witnessed in Celeste, who had approached him in another room of the clinic and said, "You are always smiling." In return, Bubby told her "You are smiling a lot too," whereupon, Celeste said, "They make those here!"

Parkinson's

Addison came to us at 77 years of age, after struggling for 11 years with Parkinson's disease. Despite being on half-a-dozen medications, his condition was deteriorating steadily. Head and bilateral hand tremors left him unable to sign his name, or eat with a fork, and made other routine tasks exceedingly difficult. He drooled when he slept; he stumbled when he walked. His inability to control his body made him embarrassed to go out in public, and the resulting social isolation left him depressed. He also complained of visual hallucinations or images that appeared in his peripheral vision, while his wife noted declines in his memory and concentration.

When Addison came to us for help, we had no idea whether BR+NAD™ would alleviate his symptoms. He'd been referred by a friend who'd undergone successful treatment for his increased use of alcohol. The friend, Charles, had been so amazed at how great he felt after his BR+NAD™ treatment that he wanted to share the treatment with everyone who might benefit. In fact, he was so convinced that BR+NAD™ could help Addison, he'd driven him to us personally. Although we'd never treated a patient with Parkinson's before, we knew that BR+NAD™ couldn't *hurt* him, so we agreed to try. It was clear to all involved that we could not make any guarantees, but with that understanding, we would certainly do all we could to help him.

We settled Addison comfortably into a reclining chair with a book, hooked him up to the intravenous drip, and went about our business attending to other patients. Addison's wife and friend Charles were sitting amiably nearby. It is customary for me to check on the rate of the intravenous drip with each patient throughout the day. About an hour after I'd started Addison's drip, I came to check on it and noticed that his elbows were resting on his legs while he read his book. Charles noticed what I was noticing and said, "Dude, your hands aren't shaking!" Addison immediately put the book down, raised his hands in front of his chest and held them up—without shaking! His wife started crying; Addison started crying; all of us in the room teared up and stared at him with gaping mouths. Walt Disney could not have done a better job of directing that scene. After two hours of treatment, Addison was able to put his book down and examine his hands at the end of his outstretched arms in total disbelief! His tremors were gone.

After six full treatments, not only were Addison's tremors gone; his peripheral hallucinations and drooling had stopped, and he no longer stumbled. A year later, he stands up straight, works out, and has even resumed riding a bike! He takes no medications other than his BR+NAD™ nasal spray. When he returned to his Parkinson's physician, she was so confounded she said, "Maybe you didn't have Parkinson's after all."

Addison has become the "poster child" for our treatment of Parkinson's disease. He comes in once a month for a maintenance dose of BR+NAD™. This is sufficient to keep all his previously exhibited symptoms at bay. He no longer drags his foot; he no longer drools; his disabling tremors are gone; no more peripheral hallucinations; and he doesn't need the c-pap to sleep. But there is more to this story. When he encounters stress his symptoms begin to reappear. When he stops using the BR+NAD™ nasal spray, there is another slight recurrence, which goes away within a few hours once he uses it. This is a direct correlation to what our Australian cohorts (see Chapter 12) have deduced: a constant supply of NAD+ is essential to proper brain functioning.

I wish I could report that all Parkinson's patients get the same amazing outcome, but that is not true. We recently treated a lovely couple from Europe. The husband was further compromised by the disease than Addison. Although there were some signs of improvement after treatment, we were not successful in meeting his goals. As with any disease, the sooner Parkinson's is detected and treated the higher the chance for a cure or remission.

Since treating Addison, we *have* treated several other patients diagnosed with some form of neurodegenerative disorder, either Parkinson's or Alzheimer's, with favorable results: the disease has either retreated or at the very least, not progressed. This is not the usual prognosis for either condition. Does BR+NAD™ turn off the epigenetic switch that had allowed the disease to advance? Does it promote effective DNA repair and neuronal energy production, both of which are decreased in Alzheimer's? In the limited number of cases we've observed, NAD+ clearly restores brain functioning; we just don't know how.

Finding out is critical. According to the Alzheimer's Association, more than 5 million Americans currently live with Alzheimer's, and one in three seniors in the U.S. dies with it or some other form of dementia. Without the development of medical breakthroughs to prevent, slow or stop the disease, the number of people age 65 and older with Alzheimer's disease could nearly triple by 2050, to as many as 130 million people.

Epidemiologic studies have shown that diet may very well play a role in neurodegenerative disorders. The rate of Alzheimer's in India, for example, is less than one-fourth what it is in the U.S. If nutritional deficiencies contribute to the development of the disease, doesn't it make sense that a nutritional supplement— NAD+—could reverse it? We are working on studies to deliver the evidence.

CTE – the football player's disease

Doug was a former college athlete—a defensive lineman— who experienced many concussions throughout his college career. At the time, however, no one called them "concussions." Instead, they'd say, he "got his bell rung." An adrenaline-fueled competitor, Doug considered his willingness to "get his bell rung" an asset; something that made him a formidable opponent on the gridiron, even though on several occasions these concussions sent him to the ICU.

Because this was before Chronic Traumatic Encephalopathy (CTE) had been identified, Doug never realized he had sustained long-term brain damage. All he knew was that now, 40 years later, he was "so amped up" all the time that he couldn't sleep. No matter how physically exhausted he was, his mind wouldn't shut off. He developed a drinking habit in order to knock himself out—literally—so that sleep could overtake him.

He knew his drinking habit wasn't healthy, but he was desperate. After passing out at night, he'd get up in the morning, take a diuretic to rid himself of the alcohol, and then complete a 30-mile bike ride in 100-degree Louisiana weather, hoping to wear himself out enough to fall asleep that night. The combination of alcohol (a dehydrator), a diuretic (another dehydrator), heat, and physical exertion finally dehydrated him to the point that a friend rushed him to St. Tammany Parish Hospital. After stabilizing him, the doctors there sent him to an alcohol rehab facility.

Doug felt that his stint in rehab was a complete waste of time. He knew *why* he drank; it wasn't to escape emotional suffering. He simply was desperate for sleep! He had no way of knowing his brain was malfunctioning because it had sustained chronic injuries as a football player.

Fortunately, another friend, our champion and former WWL radio host Garland Robinette, heard what had happened; knew that we were in the brain restoration business, so called Doug to say, "Go to Springfield Wellness Center. Paula is waiting to hear from you."

Doug, of course, was dubious. "Brain restoration"? Really? He didn't want to put himself through another treatment he didn't need. But when Doug went online to research his symptoms, he realized he was a textbook case for CTE. Of the 16 symptoms listed, Doug identified with 13:

1. Difficulty thinking (cognitive impairment)
2. Impulsive behavior
3. Depression or apathy
4. Short-term memory loss
5. Difficulty planning and carrying out tasks (executive function)
6. Emotional instability
7. Substance abuse
8. Suicidal thoughts or behavior
9. Irritability
10. Aggression
11. Speech and language difficulties

12. Vision and focusing problems
13. Trouble with sense of smell (olfactory abnormalities)

He didn't like where this was going—nor the prognosis for CTE patients. So he took Garland's advice, came to Springfield Wellness Center, and let us "hook him up."

As he says on the testimonial video he made on our behalf, "After just *20 minutes*, I felt a level of well-being and energy I hadn't felt on my own in my entire adult life. Paula and Doc and the nurses kept asking me, 'How are your cravings?' But I didn't have a *single inkling* of a craving after the first 20 minutes of the first IV.

"The medical establishment says there's no cure for CTE, but I can say with 100% sincerity, the treatment I received at Springfield Wellness Center restored my brain. I can sleep without alcohol. I'm not 'amped up' and irritable all the time. I'm not depressed. I feel great."

Although research into the etiology of CTE is ongoing, and no one can say on the basis of a single positive outcome such as Doug's that BR+NAD™ cures the disease, a single positive outcome for a condition that previously had *no* known positive outcomes is tremendously exciting. A 2015 study showed that the brains of 110 of the 111 deceased NFL football players autopsied had CTE—a horrifying 99%. And of course, professional football players aren't the only ones at risk. Youth participants in contact sports—including football, hockey, soccer, rugby, and boxing—are also vulnerable, as are the participants in these sports at the college and professional levels.

Could BR+NAD™ restore the brains of these battered athletes? Here again, we need evidence. Here is yet another reason we are investing in NAD+ studies through our foundation, NAD+Research, Inc.

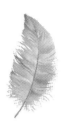

Patience and perseverance have a magical effect before
which difficulties disappear and obstacles vanish.
—John Quincy Adams

CHAPTER ELEVEN

Why Isn't This Everywhere?

"Why isn't this being used everywhere?" is a question I have been asked at every treatment rotation since 2002. Whether by patients experiencing the wonders of BR+NAD™, or loved ones who witness the brain restoration metamorphosis, someone always asks, "Why isn't this *out there*?"

For years we have been ridiculed by the very people you'd think would be banging on our door. My staff often feels dejected, but I tell them that the people "out there" do not see what we see "in here," so just wait. Those who criticize us will show up to see for themselves eventually, and when they do it will be another message from the universe to keep doing our work. We will be one step closer to our goal of making BR+NAD™ the "standard of care" for brain restoration for *many* brain-related conditions, not just addiction.

Garland Robinette, a New Orleans media icon, is an unapologetic advocate of our work. He has been instrumental in helping us get the word "out there" since first inviting us to be interviewed on his radio show after the overdose death of Whitney Houston. A mutual friend had told him that we were offering a new detox treatment with impressive results.

Following the interview, Garland called to say his telephone was lighting up as it did during Hurricane Katrina. He also told me that our greatest marketing challenge was going to be that our treatment was "too good to be true."

That is a fact. Our results are so far outside the typical results of traditional detox treatment that they have become a liability rather than an asset. Few in the medical community, especially the addiction community, can believe or accept that one little molecule, one little co-enzyme of Vitamin B3, can possibly detox a patient safely or block the cravings, or restore cognition in 10 short days. In all fairness, I would have a difficult time believing it, too, had I not seen it firsthand.

We have been criticized, in part, because medical schools still have a bias against "alternative," "complementary," "natural," "holistic," or any other name one might give to non-traditional medical practices. The notion that nutrition can be more effective in healing some diseases than pharmaceutical drugs (which come with a long list of possible side effects) is dismissed by the traditional medical establishment. My husband reports that he got two hours of nutrition education back in 1978. Today's students don't get much more. One recent graduate told us he received four hours. Why is nutrition minimized when we now have an obesity epidemic, along with heart disease, cancer, and a host of other diseases tied to diet? All diseases and disorders benefit when healthy nutrition is the foundation upon which other treatments are built. Necessary lifestyle changes are easier to make when healthy nutrition supports those transitions. Healthy nutrition can help create the energy you need to get moving, to exercise! That, too, helps you live longer!

Some critics have said that our evidence is anecdotal (I prefer to call it "clinical," and nearly 20 years' worth at this writing!) but that we lack the empirical evidence that is necessary for medical and addiction practitioners to take us seriously. There are some national addiction medicine associations, like the American

Society for Addiction Medicine (ASAM) and NAADAC (the National Association for Addiction Professionals), which now have a foothold in the mainstream medical world. They, too, are leery of endorsing a treatment that has not been medically "established," e.g., with large-scale, double-blind studies that confirm our results. Barring that, laboratory research could confirm our clinical results by identifying the mechanisms through which NAD+ works, thereby making our results plausible. Fortunately, that research is coming. We have created NAD+Research, Inc. a 501(c)(3) nonprofit entity dedicated to BR+NAD™ research. And we are not the only ones investigating the mechanisms of NAD+ functionality in the cell. More on that in Chapter 12.

In 2002, when Dr. Hitt came to cut the blue ribbon at the opening of our clinic, I invited all my friends who were in recovery to attend. To date, only one of those has recommended someone for our treatment. It has also been disheartening to have my friends who are professionals (doctors, lawyers, and others) make referrals to other programs when one of their friends or family members is in need. Fortunately, that has begun to change in the last few years. What still exists, though, are doctors and other healthcare providers who do not hide their skepticism when their patients inquire about Springfield Wellness Center and brain restoration. They will either be professional, saying something like, "I don't know enough about it to comment," or they will say something unfounded, such as, "What they claim is impossible," although they know nothing about NAD+. This, of course, dramatically reduces our physician referrals.

Imagine you admit to your doctor that you have an addiction and want to try the treatment at Springfield Wellness Center, which is an essential bio-nutrient approach to detox. It is outpatient and only takes 10 days, meaning you can return to work without having lost too much time on the job. Too often, he or she will say, "I don't think that's possible." As I write this, in 2017, we have a new physician in training who just finished his residency. He confirmed that the bias regarding "alternative" treatment is still very strong in our medical schools and residency training programs.

Fortunately, my husband and I earned respected reputations in the mental health community over the years before opening the clinic, so we have been able to weather these storms of disbelief and skepticism.

My husband, Dr. Richard Mestayer, was still on staff at the hospital when I opened the clinic in 2002. For six years I struggled, forging ahead on a wing and a prayer and a $12,000 loan from Whitney Bank. Those were tough times, but we limped along—until Hurricane Katrina. In the days before Hurricane Katrina, we had the blessing of meeting the Van Ness Butler family from Florida. Mr. and Mrs. Butler are deceased now but left a legacy of love and support for us and our mission. Along with their son, they invested in our dream at a time when it was only a dream. Without their faith and investment, I doubt we would be standing today.

There were others, too, like my friend Sue and four generous businessmen who believed and invested but, unfortunately, Katrina washed away any hope of a return on their investments.

As of May 2018, Springfield Wellness Center has treated approximately 1,500 addiction patients, while stumbling into the new territory of treating other conditions with BR+NAD™. We see evidence that the tide of acceptance is finally starting to turn in the growing number of physicians applying to be trained by BR+ MD Consultants™ and in the increased number of physicians who are making referrals for treatment.

If you ever visit us, you will see a framed letter from Ochsner Hospital, thanking Dr. Mestayer for "the fine and informative presentation of NAD+" he gave at Grand Rounds in 2013. That letter was 11 years in the making, which is why I had it framed. It is an affirmation that I value very much from an institution that I respect.

What a long, strange trip it's been

The first linkage of niacin deficiency to drug addiction was reported in the *Minerva Medica*, an Italian medical journal, in 1948 by Dr. Paolo Otenello. He published his discovery that he could painlessly detox morphine addiction with injections of vitamins, niacin, and thiamine, while most experts in the addiction field used a program of gradual reduction of the addicting substance over time. The use of a vitamin therapy alone was a radically new idea and raised questions of how it could do the job better and in less time. The answers would come later to a number of independent researchers and the tie between niacin and addiction would come into focus.

Some of the most interesting and extensive work was done by Canadian physician, biochemist, and psychiatrist Abram Hoffer, whose work linking NAD+ deficiency and schizophrenia was mentioned in Chapter 10. Dr. Hoffer was as controversial as he was critical of mainstream psychiatry. He thought biochemistry and human physiology should be the approach to solve a variety of illnesses. Fascinated with the cure for pellagra, a disease he described with "the four Ds": dermatitis, diarrhea, dementia, and death, Hoffer observed that early-stage dementia is virtually indistinguishable from schizophrenia. He theorized that mega-vitamin therapies and nutritional interventions are potentially more effective treatments for schizophrenia, alcoholism and drug addiction, cardiovascular disease, children with learning and behavioral disorders, and confused states such as dementia and memory disturbance.

Hoffer's claims regarding schizophrenia and his theories of orthomolecular medicine have been widely criticized. In 1973 the American Psychiatric Association reported methodological flaws in Hoffer's work with studies that failed to confirm the benefits of mega-vitamin treatment for treating schizophrenia.

His far-reaching theories and unconventional methods, such as conducting studies on the treatment of schizophrenia and alcoholism with LSD years before Dr. Timothy Leary, made headlines, causing an uproar in psychiatry. Some outspoken colleagues called him "arrogant" and his ideas "pure quackery." Yet Hoffer, in a 2006 interview, confidently stated that, while he believed that current mainstream psychiatric care was "terrible," his theories and treatments were starting to become more accepted. He declared "We're at a transition point. If I live another four or five years, I'll see it."[32]

Hoffer's work with schizophrenics (many of whom were alcoholics) caught the attention of Bill Wilson (Bill W.), co-founder of Alcoholics Anonymous, in 1960. As Hoffer described (Vitamin B3: Niacin and Its Amide, by A. Hoffer, M.D., Ph.D.; Wilson B: The vitamin B3 therapy: The first communication to AA's physicians (1967); A second communication to AA's physicians (1968), he and colleague Humphry Osmond introduced Wilson to the concept of mega-vitamin therapy as a potential cure for alcoholism. Wilson agreed to be a guinea pig. He began to take niacin (now known as B-3) as directed by Hoffer and, within a few weeks, the fatigue and depression that had plagued him for years were gone. Within six months he was convinced that the treatment would be very helpful to other alcoholics. Wilson gave niacin to 30 of his closest friends in AA and persuaded them to try it. Of the 30, 10 were free of anxiety, tension, and depression in one month. Another 10 were well in two months. He wanted to persuade AA members, especially the doctors, that this would be a useful addition to treatment, and he needed a term that could be readily popularized. Since the vitamin known as niacin appears third in sequencing, Wilson decided on "The Vitamin B-3 Therapy." Thousands of pamphlets

---

[32] https://robwipond.com/archives/21

were distributed under this name, and even now medical journals continue to use the term "Vitamin B-3."

However, Bill's quest became unpopular with the board members of AA International, whose medical members reportedly felt he had no business or authority recommending "medical" treatment. Although the 1960 edition of the *AA Group Handbook* included letters from AA physicians on the use of niacin to relieve alcohol addiction, in later editions those letters were omitted. It appears that Wilson had been discredited by the AA medical community, much like Hoffer by his colleagues in psychiatry. Nevertheless, RDA B-3 (much smaller doses than highly-effective mega-doses) therapy is now routinely administered to recovering addicts and alcoholics in hospitals and treatment centers, largely due to Hoffer's outside-the-box theories and Bill Wilson's efforts to incorporate mega doses of B-3 as an essential component of treatment for alcoholism.

While Wilson was working to include vitamin B-3 therapy in AA, Dr. Russell Smith carried on another early-stage investigation of niacin treatment for alcoholism. Smith was inspired by Hoffer and Osmond, treating both schizophrenics and a second group of schizophrenics afflicted with alcoholism, using very high doses of B-3 injections. The latter alcoholic group had success as a result of the treatment. Smith reported 500 schizophrenic alcoholics treated over a five-year period with success rates of 50-60%. Smith's work was largely ignored because he could not show a biochemical mechanism for his results.[33]

The 1960s further advanced NAD+ treatment specifically for alcohol and drug dependence. Over the next several decades there were a reported 22,000 addiction patients "successfully treated" with NAD+ in South Africa, although the results were never confirmed by the international scientific community,

---

[33] Smith, Russell F. Status Report Concerning the Use of Megadose Nicotinic Acid in Alcoholics, J. Orthomolecular Psychiatry, Vol. 7, No. 1: 52-55, 1978.

possibly because of the isolation of South Africa due to apartheid. Perhaps the most meaningful work during this time, however, was done by Dr. Paul O'Halloren of Shick-Shadel Hospital in Seattle. O'Halloren was the first to use the coenzyme NAD+ intravenously in addiction, closely resembling our intravenous BR+NAD™ therapy, to painlessly detox over 11,000 alcoholics and over 100 patients addicted to a variety of drugs.[34] He used the term DPN, which today is more accurately labeled as NAD+. As a result, the next generation of scientists and physicians have not always linked the two. O'Halloren prescribed NAD+ in doses of one gram per day for three days to achieve a "cure" (or favorable short-term outcome). However, relapses were common, and many addicts had to return to the hospital. Our experience at Springfield Wellness Center has taught us that the method of compounding the NAD+ is critical (the coenzyme loses potency when exposed to heat), as is a 10-day treatment regimen for most patients. O'Halloren was on the right track; his methods only needed refinement, maintenance, and behavioral therapies to achieve game-changing results.

O'Halloren developed and produced NAD+ and obtained a patent for its use in treating addiction with the support of Abbott Labs. His patent subsequently expired, however, and NAD+ therapies for addiction treatment in the U.S. thereafter disappeared...temporarily!

---

[34] O'Halloren, Paul, Diphosphopyridine Nucleotide in the Prevention, Diagnosis, and Treatment of Drug Addiction: A Preliminary Report. West. J. Surg., Obst. & Gynec., May-June 1961

The War on Drugs

For the rest of the '60s and, indeed the century, there was little advancement of NAD+ research. Then soldiers began returning from the war in Vietnam addicted to heroin. Estimates published in the *New York Times* put heroin use among American troops at 10%-25% of military personnel stationed in Southeast Asia.

President Nixon was advised to act decisively to avoid a drug and crime epidemic at home due to returning addicted soldiers. He told the country it would wage a new war, a War on Drugs and the primary weapon in this war would be methadone.

Methadone was first synthesized in 1939 Germany to address the country's short supply of opiates and was used by the Nazi military as a pain medication. Seemingly effective for wartime use, it was later thought to have little practical value because of reported side effects, including nausea and overdoses. Early subjects studied presented euphoria, inflammation of the skin, signs of toxicity, and appearance of illness. They rapidly developed a tolerance to the drug and physicians concluded that methadone carried a high potential for addiction, as well as for creating other health problems. Inexplicably, the drug still carried a non-addictive rating.[35]

After the war, German patents were distributed to the allies. U.S. pharmaceutical companies interested in the formula were able to buy the rights for commercial production for one dollar. In 1947, methadone was approved for use in the United States as an analgesic and was first manufactured by Eli Lilly under the trade name Dolophine (now registered to Roxane Labs). Mallinckrodt soon followed with its generic compound, methadone.

It wasn't until studies performed at the Rockefeller Foundation by Vincent Dole, Marie Nyswander, and Mary

---

[35] http://www.narconon.org/drug-information/methadone-history.html

Jeanne Kreek that methadone was systematically studied as a potential substitution therapy. These researchers believed that long-term heroin use caused a permanent metabolic deficiency in the central nervous system and an associated physiological disease that required ongoing indefinite dosing of opiates to correct this metabolic deficiency, much like daily insulin injections for diabetics. Dole's Rockefeller conclusions published 50 years ago have been embraced worldwide, and methadone maintenance therapy (MMT) remains the gold standard today.[36]

Similar to the American Medical Association's 1956 declaration that alcoholism was an illness, Dole's studies began a sweeping change in the notion that drug addiction was not necessarily a character flaw, but a disorder to be treated in the same way as other diseases. Critics of methadone maintenance therapy agree that drug addiction is a disease but treating the addiction should be the approach rather than treating a metabolic deficiency. This debate rages on today with newer opioid replacement therapies.

To date, methadone maintenance therapy (MMT) has been the most politically polarizing of any pharmacotherapy for the treatment of drug addiction patients. The industry claims it is the most systematically studied and boasts success rates of 60-90%; however, looking behind the numbers raises questions. *Harvard Health* reports, "It has been estimated that 25% of patients eventually become abstinent, 25% continue to take the drug, and 50% go on and off methadone repeatedly."[37]

The 25% of patients free from dependence on opioids certainly points to some success, and the 25% remaining on methadone maintenance (presumably until death) is counted

[36] http://centennial.rucares.org/index.php?page=Methadone_Maintenance

[37] Treating opiate addiction, Part I: Detoxification and maintenance, Harvard Health Publishing, April 2005.
https://www.health.harvard.edu/mind-and-mood/treating-opiate-addiction-part-i-detoxification-and-maintenance

as a success under the MMT model adopted 50 years ago. The remaining 50% going "on and off methadone repeatedly" offers little insight into recidivism, natural death, homicide, suicide, overdose, and lengths of abstinence.

The methadone maintenance industry, supervised and sanctioned by government agencies like Substance Abuse Mental Health Services Administration (SAMHSA), claims only minor side effects from methadone, which may include shallow breathing, lightheadedness, rash or swelling of the face, lips, or tongue, nausea, and sedation. Treatment industry giant, CRC Health, which was recently acquired by Acadia and owns more than 100 clinics, reports similar benign side effects for methadone maintenance. Although the literature is not clear as to whether or not methadone is an easier withdrawal than other opioids, physicians trained in addiction medicine, along with methadone users themselves, agree that prolonged methadone use at high doses makes withdrawal nearly impossible without long-term hospitalization. NIDA studies show that methadone maintenance is most effective at durations of at least one year and dosages of at least 75 milligrams.[38]

Studies conducted at Castle Craig Hospital in Edinburg, the heroin capital of the UK, boldly point out dangers and health risks not embraced by the methadone treatment industry in the United States.[39] They report methadone is responsible for 25% of opioid deaths and that treatment duration more than eight months renders most addicts unmotivated to become drug-free. The study, spanning 30 years, determined that methadone directly causes malnourishment and osteoporosis, causing bones to fracture easily and teeth to fall out, and also causes changes in brain chemistry resulting in mood disorders and diminished cognitive functioning. Any notion that methadone users can return to a normal life under such physical and chemical trauma is unfounded,

---

[38] https://www.drugabuse.gov/sites/default/files/pdf/partb.pdf
[39] www.livestrong.com/article/209186-long-term-effects-from-methadone-use/

substantiated by many physicians and former methadone users themselves. Furthermore, Castle Craig's 30-year study found that methadone programs prolong an addict's injecting career from 5 to 30 years, which is contrary to any research and literature of the methadone industry in the United States.

Henry Pierce, CEO of Federal City Recovery Centers in Washington DC, has been working with heroin addicts for the last 30 years. Pierce, a recovering heroin addict himself, was once on a methadone maintenance program of 100 mg daily, and when he made the decision to detox, he was told at the clinic that he couldn't be taken off treatment because of the high dosage (a dosage which was protocol under federal guidelines). Rather than a "life sentence" of poor health and daily visits to methadone clinics, Pierce said his only alternative was to begin using heroin again to detox from the methadone and then to suffer heroin withdrawal symptoms, which were less severe. In his residential treatment programs, Pierce carefully screens incoming addicts and says his methadone populations are "physically compromised," adding, "they suffer from depression and are emotionally unresponsive, making recovery very difficult." Another long-time addiction specialist, co-founder of an inpatient treatment center serving high poverty communities, echoes Pierce's observations, calling methadone, "just another form of chemical slavery."

SAMHSA's guidelines for dispensing methadone at an opioid treatment facility are claimed to be reasonable, and they say treatment is safe and effective if taken as prescribed; however, methadone, being a full agonist, can and will be abused. According to the CDC in 2012 methadone accounted for nearly one-third of opioid deaths and in 82% of those cases reported by the U.S. National Center for Health Statistics, involved combining methadone with other drugs.

Suburban America has a heroin problem

In the 40 years following the federal government's inaugural sponsorship of methadone clinics, heroin use in the United States has climbed to over 1,000,000 users, which is three times the number of heroin users in 2003, says the UN Office on Drugs and Crime upon release of its 2016 World Drug Report. Even more shocking is that reported deaths related to heroin use have increased five-fold since 2000. These statistics are consistent with DEA reports for the same periods.

The rise in heroin addiction is not a mystery. Twenty years ago, new pain management therapies were introduced, and it is widely accepted that these medications were overprescribed. The DEA discovered that millions of patients were relying on drugs such as OxyContin, Vicodin, Percocet or Lortab for relief from severe pain but also became addicted. Overdoses were common, with media coverage reducing physicians and pharmaceutical company CEOs to drug traffickers, singling out Purdue Pharma's OxyContin as more harmful than heroin. Under pressure, the federal government expanded supervision and imposed restrictions on distribution, and the FDA elevated hydrocodone combination drugs to Schedule II narcotics in 2013. By this time, addiction was so entrenched that demand went underground, to illicit prescription traffickers who produced inexpensive counterfeits containing fentanyl. The Centers for Disease Control (CDC) reported in 2016 that deaths in 2014 from synthetic opioids like fentanyl showed an increase of 80%,[40] while the NIH reported that 10 million Americans, 4.1% of the adult population, used opioid painkillers for nonmedical reasons in 2014. In a new environment of rigorous federal and state prescription monitoring programs and increasing demand for painkillers, the deep and vast heroin and fentanyl markets

---

[40] https://www.cdc.gov/mmwr/preview/mmwrhtml/mm6450a3.htm

readily absorbed displaced addicts seeking a drug that's easier to get, easier to use, and easier to afford. The price of heroin in 1980, with an average retail-level purity of 10%, was $3,260 per gram. By 2007, one gram of heroin in the retail market cost $131, the lowest price since UN records began in 1990, according to *The Economist*.[41] But what is also striking about the current epidemic is its location in suburban areas and outlying counties, rather than inner cities as was the case in the 1960s, 1970s, and 1980s.

Buprenorphine drugs: an opioid shell game

In 1969 researchers at Reckitt & Colman (now Reckitt Benckiser) spent 10 years attempting to synthesize an opioid compound "with structures substantially more complex than morphine that could retain the desirable actions while shedding the undesirable side effects."[42] What they came up with was an effective alternative to morphine, called buprenorphine, a partial agonist with a very slow onset that led the researcher to conclude that the drug would be safer and less likely to be abused. Buprenorphine was first launched in the UK as an injection for chronic pain. A sublingual formulation was released in 1982.

Reckitt Benckiser recognized both the blossoming opioid epidemic and the dangers associated with methadone maintenance and, challenging the methadone industry, lobbied the United States Congress to authorize the Secretary of Health & Human Services to grant waivers to approved physicians to administer buprenorphine drugs for opioid detox

---

[41] http://www.economist.com/node/13917432

[42] (Campbell N. D.; Lovell A. M. (2012) The history of the development of buprenorphine as an addiction therapeutic." *Annals of the New York Academy of Sciences*. 1248: 124–139)

and maintenance therapies. The resulting Drug Addiction Treatment Act of 2000 permitted the use of Reckitt Benckiser's buprenorphine, branded Subutex, which trades as Buprenex and Cizdol under other manufacturers. Currently, the treatment of choice for opioid addiction outpatient settings is Suboxone, which is buprenorphine with naloxone (antagonist) manufactured by Indivior, a Reckitt Benckiser subsidiary. Suboxone is the most widely prescribed buprenorphine drug.

Suboxone, with properties of both partial agonist and opiate blocker, was eagerly received upon FDA approval in 2002. Suboxone's primary advantage is an elimination half-life almost double that of methadone's, which means users don't have to take a dose daily. The potential for overdose, abuse, and addiction is considered to be less with Suboxone because of its partial agonist status, which introduces a ceiling effect. Also, according to manufacturers, the naloxone will cause unpleasant symptoms if snorted or injected.

Suboxone was believed to be much harder to abuse so is available by prescription through a physician that has met federal requirements, whereas methadone is known to be commonly abused and patients must travel to a clinic at least once, sometimes twice per day, to obtain it. Suboxone literature claims it is less addictive, withdrawal symptoms are less severe, and risk of fatal overdose on Suboxone is less than with methadone. However, as with methadone maintenance therapy, there is a lack of credible long-term studies on Suboxone maintenance.

Former NIDA director, Dr. Alan Leshner, speaking to the *New York Times* in 2004, described buprenorphine drugs as "the most important advance certainly in heroin and opiate treatment, if not all addiction treatments, in the last 30 years," a statement with which few in the treatment industry disagree. However, clinicians remain sharply divided as to whether Suboxone should be used for maintenance therapy (theoretically displacing methadone), or used as a tool to detox addicts from opioids.

Popular treatment industry website, *The Fix*, featured a 2011 story by Jennifer Matesa highlighting both champions and critics of Suboxone maintenance.[43] Dr. Jeffrey Junig, a psychiatrist in Fond du Lac, Wisconsin and professor of psychiatry at the Medical College of Wisconsin, has a private practice treating opiate addiction with buprenorphine maintenance. He maintains his client base at the federal limit of 100 (amended in 2016 to a maximum of 275). Junig aggressively uses media such as blogs, websites and YouTube videos to promote maintenance therapy and tear down stigmas he says exist surrounding medication-assisted therapies. However, Matesa writes that his advocacy of buprenorphine maintenance is based on "least-worst" logic, noting that, if patients terminate treatment or merely taper off, they return to active addiction. Consequently, Junig recommends buprenorphine maintenance for life.

Critics of Suboxone maintenance are easily found. In the same article by Matesa in *The Fix*, she quotes Dr. Stephen Scanlan, director of Palm Beach Outpatient Detox in the heart of Florida's "pill-mill" country, where he says more than two-thirds of the nation's oxycodone prescriptions are written. Scanlan, board certified in psychiatry, neurology and addiction medicine, is a recovered addict himself, becoming addicted to opiates when he was a resident in anesthesiology. Ironically, he credits buprenorphine for saving his life and the lives of thousands he has treated, calling it "the most amazing detox tool I've ever seen." However, Scanlan is a fierce opponent of maintenance therapy that keeps patients on the drug for months or years. While his average detox using Suboxone is 20-25 days for heroin, pharma drugs like OxyContin, and even methadone, he says withdrawal from long-term Suboxone use is extraordinarily difficult and must be done by a physician trained in addiction medicine. Scanlan claims that detox from Suboxone will take

---

[43] https://www.thefix.com/content/best-kept-secret-addiction-treatment?page=all

4-5 months (sometimes as long as a year for long-term high-dose users), incorporating 10 different medications. He explained in an article titled *Detoxing from Suboxone—Fear is Caused by a Lack of Knowledge*, that "the problem I am finding in America is that doctors know how to get patients on Suboxone but no one knows how to get them off it," adding that the large majority of these physicians prescribing Suboxone have "no training in addiction medicine." According to the SAMSHA website, a physician can be granted a waiver to prescribe buprenorphine drugs simply by attending an 8-hour online training and passing a post-test.

As you can imagine, I have a hard time reading accounts like this without being beside myself with frustration.

The pharmaceutical industry's claims that Suboxone's abuse potential is low and that it doesn't present any mental or physical health problems is "just false advertising" according to Scanlan, quoted again by Matesa in *The Fix*. The naloxone doesn't prevent the addict from withdrawal and Suboxone *can* be shot intravenously and snorted. Moreover, it is commonly sold on the street, according to scores of Scanlan's patients. Curiously, there are no long-term studies on Suboxone maintenance, but doctors have identified health problems in this population identical to symptoms found in long-term methadone users. Scanlan says, "I've seen what long-term Suboxone does. People come in with endocrine problems, thyroid dysfunction, low testosterone, which kills sex drive, hair loss, and even tooth loss." The notion that Suboxone maintenance gives time for the addict's damaged brain to heal is quickly dismissed by Scanlan: "There's no way brain chemistry can heal while on buprenorphine. You're continuing to give someone a narcotic." This is consistent with our experience with BR+NAD™. Switching from one opiate—whether heroin or methadone—to another (Suboxone) does not heal the neurological aspect of addiction, which is characterized in part by the phenomenon of tolerance: as long as exogenous opioids are taken, the body decreases its production of endorphins.[44]

Scanlan's claims that Suboxone can and will be abused are consistent with other addiction experts on the front lines. Percy Menzies, pharmacist/addiction expert and president of Assisted Recovery Centers of America, says plainly, "Buprenorphine is one of the most abused pharmaceuticals in the world." The problem with Suboxone, according to Menzies, "is that many addicts have learned they can use the medication, not to treat their addiction, but to maintain it. Suboxone won't get them 'high,' but it will help them smooth out withdrawal symptoms between highs."

Buprenorphine drug Suboxone is so popular with addicts that it has turned into a street drug that can be exchanged for money, heroin or other drugs.[45] Law enforcement estimates that about half of the buprenorphine obtained through legitimate prescriptions is either being diverted or used illicitly. "We joke that there's more Suboxone on the street than in pharmacies. Heroin dealers are diversified now. They offer a choice of Suboxone and heroin. And with all these generic forms coming out, that is going to explode," says Menzies. "We took an abused drug, and we said let's use it to treat addiction to heroin and opiates." (ibid)

NAD+ Hitts the 21st Century

During the last 20 years of the 20th century, intravenous NAD+ therapies finally gained traction, as I mentioned, with the work of Dr. William Hitt in Mexico. Picking up the mantle of non-narcotic brain restoration therapy after Dr. Hitt's death,

---

[44] https://www.ncbi.nlm.nih.gov/pmc/articles/PMC3104618/
[45] http://nationalpainreport.com/suboxone-new-drug-epidemic-8821747.html

we at Springfield Wellness Center have been leading the way with intravenous BR+NAD™ therapy in the U.S. since 2001.

A national emergency missing the mark

In October 2017, the President of the United States declared the nation's opioid epidemic a national emergency. Accordingly, billions of dollars will be invested in tackling this public health problem. *Virtually none* of that money is likely to be invested in a medical treatment model that can *quickly, safely,* and *effectively* detox addiction patients *without substituting another narcotic,* while restoring their brains to healthy functioning, with all the benefits that implies. Needless to say, I find that extremely frustrating—and indeed, tragic.

One year ago today I wrote the chapter called Veterans Day. So much has happened since writing that chapter, but I pause again this Veterans Day to add a message I hope will be embraced by the military community on ALL levels.

We must "inform and encourage" not only the precious souls who are afflicted with the scourge of addiction but also those in positions of influence who can certainly make a difference—not only for veterans but others in need. Where are all the insurance companies that could help their clients with a treatment of unrivaled effectiveness and unprecedented detoxification and brain restoration treatment? Where are all the philanthropic billionaires who could not only fund our veterans' treatment but could fund the research that would verify our clinical results and help make our treatment "the standard of care." I watch the news seeing all the beautiful gifts and programs given to the veterans from very thoughtful and generous wealthy individuals and corporations. I hope someone is listening and will at least send a scout or envoy to Springfield Wellness Center to see whether we are legitimate. I can assure you we are. No one has walked through the doors of Springfield Wellness Center without walking out saying, "Why isn't this available everywhere?"

One veteran who has been in treatment with us for the last few months came in with post-traumatic stress so severe that his anxiety literally drove his life. On one occasion during a counseling session, he was able to let go and actually cry. He hid his face, and when he looked up and saw the tears running down my face, too, said, "I've never had a doctor cry with me before!" That was the magical bonding moment. He is still soldiering up, and we are moving forward, but our progress is slow because he doesn't have the insurance or financial means to pay for intravenous BR+NAD™ treatment. If he had the insurance or funds, or if we still had money in our fundraising reserved for veterans, he would be free today. Instead, we persevered with the slower titrating protocols, which include delivering BR+NAD™ through other mechanisms—nasal spray, patches, cream, and sub-cutaneous shots.

This is heartbreaking to me. Please listen: I'm a clinician with nearly 40 years of experience—nearly half of them advocating for BR+NAD™. I'm one tiny voice screaming in this collective "dark night of the soul," pleading for attention because what we do *works*.

I've sent letters to many famous and influential people. I realize that they may not have even seen the letters, but now that we have a declared national emergency I pray that someone with influence will read this book. Our treatment not only helps those with addiction, but also people with other conditions resulting from traumatic brain injury, environmental toxins, concussions, and the aging process. I don't claim our work will "cure" anyone, but I can tell you that our work offers hope to everyone. With the proper support, we *will* find "cures" where there are none now. It is just a matter of time. "And money," quips Billy, our own 007!

We call Billy "007" because he was the 7th patient I treated and the one who calls me *every* September 9th, his birthday, to thank me for saving his life. Billy is my buddy and my crusader. He sends me a steady stream of new information that crosses his path via the web and social media. He protects me and our mission. I am very grateful for the wise and encouraging counsel he has given me over the years when I felt defeated. He constantly reminds me not to forget his brothers in the "hood" who also need this treatment, I haven't and I won't! Hopefully, this book will help me keep that promise.

Billy has seen me through some tough times. He is a thoughtful and compassionate soul. When I told him my mother died in my arms and that an indescribable blanket of Peace and Grace descended upon my sister and me, he said, "Oh Paula, just think about it. You took your first breath with her and she took her last breath with you."

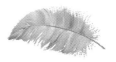

We cannot solve our problems with the same thinking we used when we created them.
—Albert Einstein

CHAPTER TWELVE

On The Hunt for
Empirical Evidence

So, what is this molecule with the power to heal? How does it work? Where does it come from and how important is it? Why do we see such remarkable, "too good to be true" outcomes with our patients? What do we need to convince the skeptics and be embraced by the American Medical Association?

Empirical evidence! Large-scale, double-blind studies, or peer-accepted, reproducible laboratory results showing the one or more mechanisms by which NAD+ works to restore the brain. These are the keys that unlock the door to credibility within the international medical establishment.

Fortunately, and at long last, this evidence is coming—building upon a foundation laid down by researchers more than 100 years ago.

On January 26, 1907, a baby was born in Vienna, Austria-Hungary, who became a world-renowned endocrinologist. His investigations led him to coin the term "stress," which is now a common household word. His name was Hans Selye, and I was introduced to his work during my internship in graduate school. What I remember most from those days is that, as a young medical resident in Canada, Dr. Selye noticed something interesting about all the patients in the hospital. Irrespective of their "diagnosis," he observed that people had similar symptoms. He first described the similarities as "noxious agents," which he later referred to as "stress." He developed a theory of stress he called the "general adaptation syndrome," which was foundational to his work on biological stress. Dr. Selye noticed that stress was different from other physical responses because stress induces biochemical changes in the body regardless of whether the stressor is good or bad, positive or negative. Dr. Selye called positive stress (getting married, giving birth, or winning the lottery, for example) "eustress" and negative stress he called "distress." Both kinds involve the hypothalamic-pituitary-adrenal axis (HPA axis), which governs how the body copes with stress. He identified three ascending stress states: the "alarm state," the "resistance state," and the "exhaustion state." (You don't want to spend a lot of time in the "exhaustion state" because the next state is death!)

It's clear that stress has become an even greater health issue today than it was in the early 1900s when Dr. Selye was writing, lecturing, and researching the stresses of life. That's because, for most people, the stress of modern living is constant—and the human body did not evolve to handle constant stress. As a result, the body's normal ability to deal with occasional stress situations is being overwhelmed, and a new illness precursor has been identified: *oxidative stress*.

Oxidative stress is a term to describe an imbalance to cellular structure that exceeds the body's ability to repair. In most cases, oxidative stress is caused by reactive oxygen species (ROS) free radicals, which, at low levels perform essential cellular functions. However, the overproduction of ROS can damage DNA, proteins, and fats, which promotes aging and the development of diseases ranging from cancer to dementia.

Oxidative stress also appears to be a major factor in the disease we call addiction.

Years ago, while in my internship, I saw a documentary showing what happens to the brain of cocaine addicts when shown a variety of pictures on a computer screen while fastened to cranial electrodes. This was *new* science at the time because being able to see the functionality of the brain was now possible and it was a big deal. It made a strong impression on me for two reasons: one, because we could actually see the brain respond, and two, because of how dramatically the brain responded. Seeing people with electrodes on their heads calmly watching benign images of flowers, birds, ocean views, a car, a boat, etc. was interesting only because of what happened when an occasional line of cocaine, or a needle, or other drug paraphernalia was randomly shown. Shockingly, the midbrain of each participant lit up like a flashlight! What did *that* mean?

I recently watched a lecture given by Dr. Kevin McCauley that I found very helpful.[46] His presentation was entertaining and informative, which is always advantageous for attention-deficit sufferers like me. He was addressing the disease model of addiction, which was first embraced by the American Medical Association in 1956. That was a long time ago, but I can tell you from my clinical experience that the needle hasn't moved much in a positive direction since then. Here we are, 61 years later, and we are still debating whether addiction is a "choice" or a "disease."

Dr. McCauley humorously and logically presented his defense of the "disease" model, which interestingly centers on the midbrain.

What constitutes a disease? Dr. McCauley presented the 100-plus-year old medical model of disease as having an organ, having a defect, having symptoms, and a cause. One dictionary defines disease as an incorrectly functioning organ

---

[46] https://www.youtube.com/watch?v=b2emgrRoT2c

or system of the body having a defect with symptoms caused by genetics, infections, poisons, nutritional deficiency, toxicity, or environmental factors or illness. Before this medical model was used, the doctor would spend a lot of time focusing on the symptoms, which might or might not respond to treatment because the "cause" of the defect was not first identified. The symptoms could span numerous diseases so knowing the "cause" helps in diagnosing and treatment.

Choice vs. Disease

In the debate between "choice" vs. "disease" in addiction medicine, a distinction needs to be made between "behaviors" vs. "symptoms." The "choice" model argues that addiction cannot be a disease because it is caused by behavior and behavior is a "choice." The "disease" model argues that the symptoms are not *actually* a choice, but the result of a biological impairment to the midbrain. Just as a diabetic cannot change his or her blood-sugar level at will, an addict cannot stop craving at will. In the diabetic, the body's inability to produce or effectively utilize insulin is the cause. In the addict, improper functioning of the midbrain is the cause. Both diseases produce symptoms that can cause unwanted behaviors. But as my friend and colleague, Dr. Liz Stuller, emphasizes to her residents in training, "You must find the root cause if you are going to successfully treat a patient. Identify the root cause!"

McCauley's definition of addiction is, "The dysregulation of the midbrain dopamine system due to unmanaged stress resulting in symptoms of decreased functioning—specifically loss of control, cravings, and persistent drug use despite negative consequences."

Although there are other organs involved in addiction, like

the liver, pancreas, and more, the brain is our focus because this is where we will find the root cause. Addiction is first a brain disease and here is why.

The prefrontal cortex is associated with what we call "executive" functions like reasoning, abstract thought, self-control, planning and organization, emotional meaning such as love, and morality, spirituality, ethics, and responsibility. Some consider it the "seat of the self," where personality and conscious awareness reside. Interestingly, *drugs don't work in the prefrontal cortex*; they work in the midbrain. This was first demonstrated by a series of experiments conducted in the '60s called the Olds Experiments, in which a probe the diameter of a hair was used to determine which area of the brain was affected by drug use (specifically, the drug cocaine). The Olds Experiments inserted probes to every possible region of the brain of rats, but the areas that resulted in addictive behavior—continual self-administration of additional doses of the drug—were the lateral hypothalamus, the nucleus accumbens, and the ventral tegmental areas (VTA) of the midbrain. Test animals would work continuously—lever-pressing at rates of several thousand responses per hour—for days to obtain direct electrical stimulation of the lateral hypothalamus and related brain regions.[47]. The animals did so to the exclusion of other behaviors, starving themselves for the opportunity to self-stimulate if food and stimulation were concurrently available for only a limited portion of each day. (ibid, Routtenberg and Lindy, 1965) Once experienced with the stimulation, rats would cross electrified grids to gain access to the lever, accepting higher shocks to obtain stimulation than they were willing to accept to obtain food, even when deprived for 24 hours. (ibid, Olds, 1959) (What person familiar with addiction doubts this result?)

Subsequent research has demonstrated that not only rats,

---

[47] Olds 1958b, Annau et al. 1974

http://www.cell.com/neuron/pdf/S0896-6273(02)00965-0.pdf

but monkeys as well, will work similarly compulsively for intravenous stimulants to the midbrain. If given unlimited access, they will self-administer intravenous injections of these drugs to the point of severe weight loss and death. (ibid, Johanson et al. 1976, Bozarth and Wise 1985) What begins as a tentative response tendency becomes a compulsive habit very quickly.[48]

The drug apparently convinces the midbrain that obtaining more of the drug is more important than anything and everything. *The drug becomes tantamount to survival.*

That's because the midbrain is where your survival instinct resides. Your midbrain is unconscious and reacts to sensory information all day, every day. It processes the life or death signaling messages, with the fight-flight-or-freeze mechanism on stand-by. These are the areas where addiction is processed, *not* the prefrontal cortex. The midbrain is also where reward and pleasure are processed. Addiction causes a defect in the midbrain long before the prefrontal cortex is affected. In fact, when the midbrain is activated to go into survival mode, it shuts down the prefrontal cortex. Brain imaging studies have shown this: when the midbrain is lit up, the prefrontal cortex is dark.

The tendency to label an addict or an alcoholic by the behaviors they exhibit while "under the influence" is understandable. If you have been on the receiving end of that behavior, without having the awareness or restraint to keep from lashing out with labels such as selfish, lying, cheating, stealing, criminal, sociopathic, entitled brat, loser, and "in denial," then welcome to the human race. Unfortunately, that type of interaction only makes matters worse. Why? Because the addict's prefrontal cortex has been high-jacked by the midbrain. To the non-addicted, those of us with access to the executive functioning of the prefrontal cortex, it's absolutely clear what addicts need to do: change their

---

[48] Wise, Roy A. Brain Reward Circuitry: Review Insights from Unsensed Incentives, Neuron, Vol. 36, 229–240, October 10, 2002, Cell Press.
http://www.cell.com/neuron/pdf/S0896-6273(02)00965-0.pdf

behavior. But as a practical medical matter, the only way an addict can successfully use the prefrontal cortex to address his or her addiction is by first addressing the defect in the midbrain. Moreover, I question the therapeutic value of labeling someone an addict or alcoholic when the label carries such negative connotations—generating guilt, shame, insecurity, and self-doubt. These, in turn, spark anxiety, depression, insomnia, and fatigue—increasing the stress that, in the addict's brain, can only be relieved by drugs. Dopamine gets the credit for relieving stress and the blame when addiction neutralizes the dopamine response, but there are other neurotransmitters like glutamine, serotonin, GABA and some we haven't yet discovered that may also be involved. Moreover, there is some data to suggest that NAD+ itself may function as a neurotransmitter, implying that if NAD+ levels are low, the addicted patient is further prevented from stress relief. However, this warrants further examination.

Stress? We ALL have stress!

Critics of the disease model of addiction like to say that stress comes in different sizes: severe, traumatic, chronic, moderate, or mild. Stress changes the physiology of the midbrain. We each experience stress differently depending on our coping mechanisms, some of which are hereditable—the genetic and epigenetic ones. However, above a certain threshold that is unique to each individual, the midbrain processes stress as a threat to survival, commanding the body to remain in constant "fight-flight-or-freeze" mode until dopamine, the body's stress-reliever, is released, which enables it to relax. An addict has learned to get that dopamine release from a drug. That strategy makes sense because an addicted brain's dopamine-production ability has been shut down—by the drug.

For those addicted to opiates or other painkillers, the same dynamic functions with endorphins, the body's natural painkiller. The brain's production capacity has been replaced by the drug, leaving a single pathway to pain relief: the narcotic. (A secondary reason for an addict to seek a drug is to get relief from excruciating withdrawals.)

The truth is that being under the influence of a substance is not limited only to the state of intoxication. *A person is still under the influence of the drug even after they sober up because their brain is still impaired.* The midbrain continues to insist that survival is at stake, and only a dopamine release will change that. At this point, addicts are no longer seeking to get "high," but to relieve the agony produced by stress and the cortisol-releasing factor (CRF) in the midbrain. In fact, the limited success of most drug treatment programs is based on substituting one (legal) drug for the illegal one that has caused the addiction in the first place. Whether the replacement drug is methadone, Suboxone, caffeine, nicotine, or sugar, its biochemical role is the same: to quiet the midbrain with a dopamine release. Twelve-step programs like AA and NA attempt to augment biochemical coping strategies with social and emotional support—because these, too, reduce anxiety. But none of them do what BR+NAD™ appears to do: reset the brain to its pre-addicted state.

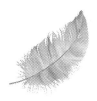

It isn't what we don't know that gives us trouble;
it's what we know that ain't so.
—Will Rogers

NAD+ The missing link

So why is the addict's brain different from a non-addicted brain?

Let's have a look at how science is beginning to explain the results we see at Springfield Wellness Center—and others who have adopted our methods—have seen clinically. The information I'm presenting here is based on information gathered and woven together in collaboration with our Australian partners (Drs. Ross Grant, Jade Berg, and Nady Braidy) and Dr. James Watson in Los Angeles. For those readers who may not remember much of their biochemistry, or who had good reasons not to take it at all, let me begin by saying that a diagram of the Krebs cycle alone is enough to trigger medical school anxiety flashbacks in Dr. Mestayer. After taking that dreaded first test—a biochemistry test—one student left campus never to be seen again, one went hysterically blind for about 30 minutes, and one passed out. So, let's take this slowly.

Dr. James Watson is a well-respected plastic surgeon on the clinical faculty of UCLA Medical School. He also is the author of a website and blog on the molecular biology of aging.[49] When he learned of our work with NAD+, he contacted us. That contact led to a deep friendship, as well as a powerful professional relationship. As a result, Dr. Watson became one of the keynote speakers at our first 2015 Brain Restoration Summit. Why? Because Dr. Watson is convinced that the same processes that leads to the death of cells, the overwhelming of the body's stress response systems, and the degeneration associated with aging, are also implicated in the disease of addiction.

In his Summit presentation, Dr. Watson outlined three factors responsible for addiction. Two may be considered hereditable: genetics (DNA), which can confer greater sensibility to various environmental factors, including alcohol

---

[49] www.Anti-agingFirewalls.com

and drugs; and epigenetics (DNA regulation), which, although also influenced by non-hereditable factors, turn gene expression off and on. Epigenetic changes in gene expression do not invoke changes to the underlying DNA sequence; rather, epigenetics determine when genes are active or inactive. (In other words, changes to phenotype, rather than genotype.) Whether the genes are active or inactive affects how cells read the genes in response to various environmental factors.

Research has identified a number of genes that, if turned on, become risk factors for addiction: one is responsible for the brain's "reward" pathway; another is responsible for ethanol (alcohol) stimulation, while a third is responsible for ethanol (alcohol) depression. There is also a "relief" pathway gene and many more.

Although epigenetic change is a common and essential occurrence governing processes such as the instructions for cells to differentiate into blood cells, brain cells, or skin cells, for example, epigenetics can also be influenced by factors such as age, disease, stress, and drug use, to result in diseases like cancer, chronic inflammation, psychiatric disorders, and many more, including addiction.

The third factor in addiction is environmental. Environmental variables include pollutants, physical activity, alcohol, and drugs. For example, the regular intake of fruit and vegetables and regular physical activity result in positive epigenetic changes; whereas regular alcohol consumption, trauma, toxins, illness, or chronic stress adversely impacts a number of genetic switches. These adverse environmental exposures can be summarized in a single word, *stress*.

Genetic and epigenetic factors alone do not cause addiction, as Dr. Watson emphasized at our Summit. Environmental factors alone do not cause addiction. But the three can come together to result in addiction due to the functioning of a single molecule: **NAD+**

NAD+ plays a critical role in all three addiction risk factors.

It repairs DNA, which can be damaged by oxidative stress, including drug use. It restores healthy epigenetic functioning—the turning off of epigenetic risk factors related to addiction. And it restores the brain to healthy functioning—including dopamine and endorphin production—so that the addict doesn't need a drug to get midbrain relief. Watson calls this the Gene-Environmental Interaction, or GEI or GXE. The environmental factor of oxidative stress triggers the epigenetic factor to turn on the expression of the genetic factor (DNA).

Watson notes that NAD+ is not the only epigenetic mechanism at the body's disposal, but it *is* involved in several of the pathways implicated in addiction. And his analysis also sheds light on how and why intravenous NAD+ given to patients suffering from addiction or withdrawal yields such positive results: it starts to return the body to its normal, healthy functioning, with positive genes turned on, and negative genes turned off. Also, it helps the body right the oxidative stress imbalance, repairing DNA and fueling mitochondrial energy production.

Another research team, led by Corinne Lasmézas, underscored the importance of NAD+ in DNA repair. Lasmézas and colleagues (2015) at the Scripps Research Institute[50] in Jupiter, Florida, and reported in *ALS Forum*, showed that depletion of NAD+, a metabolite necessary for energy production, drives neuronal death. Research compiled at the Linus Pauling Institute, Oregon State University, summarizes some of the various implications of niacin—and its precursor, NAD+—deficiency.[51] Disease states impacted by niacin and

[50] Minghai Zhou Gregory OttenbergGian Franco Sferrazza Christopher HubbsMohammad Fallahi Gavin RumbaughAlicia F. Brantley Corinne I. Lasmézas, Neuronal death induced by misfolded prion protein is due to NAD⁺ depletion and can be relieved *in vitro* and *in vivo* by NAD⁺ replenishment, Brain, Volume 138, Issue 4, 1 April 2015, Pages 992–1008, https://doi.org/10.1093/brain/awv002

[51] Linus Pauling Institute Micronutrient Information Center, Niacin http://lpi.oregonstate.edu/mic/vitamins/niacin

nicotinamide deficiency range from pellagra to schizophrenia to prevention of cancer to reduction of the risk of cardiac arrest. Most notably, "NAD+ is the sole substrate for PARP enzymes involved in DNA repair activity in response to DNA strand breaks; thus, NAD+ is critical for genome stability," the Oregon State researchers note.

In the same video of Dr. Kevin McCauley referenced above, he also shares some stunning information related to the epigenetics of babies born to mothers who had been abused during their first trimester.[52] The mothers had a significantly greater chance of giving birth to babies who grow up having problems with anger, ADHD (attention-deficit hyperactivity disorder), addiction to stimulants, and chronic stress such as undiagnosed mental illness. In other words, the stress-induced changes to the epigenetics of the mothers were passed on to their babies. Over time, these conditions cause hormonal changes (increased production of corticotropin-releasing factor, or CRF) to the midbrain because the stress is constant; it simply does not go away.

Anhedonia is a psychiatric term for patients who are no longer able to find pleasure from things they found pleasurable in the past. The result is that once there is a new dopamine rush from chemicals like alcohol, sedatives, opiates, cocaine, amphetamines, hallucinogens, steroids, nicotine, caffeine, inhalants, or cannabinoids, the drug becomes the new coping mechanism for all incoming stressors! Simply put, stress creates cravings and, as I mentioned before, an addict cannot choose not to crave. Millions of people have attended AA meetings to stave off acting on the craving for just another hour. Some last an hour and 10 minutes, some 10 more hours, some 10 days, and some 10 years or more. All suffer from each passing minute until, or unless, their recovery management plan brings them a miracle or the healing they are desperate to find.

---

[52] https://www.youtube.com/watch?v=b2emgrRoT2c

Springfield Wellness Center is recognized for having done the most clinical research on IV NAD+ in the United States, refining the NAD+ formula for effective patient detox. Our trademarked BR+NAD™ 10-day addiction detox has been used to treat over 1,500 people with success. Moreover, the protocol reduces withdrawal symptoms by 70%-80% without using addictive replacement drugs. Most patients report clarity and well-being to pre-use levels and typically leave our facility without the need for *any* additional medications.

Our dear friend and colleague, Dr. Ross Grant, of the University of New South Wales School of Medical Sciences, has published 50 papers on NAD+ metabolism. Grant's research focuses on aging and oxidative stress, a process involving free radical damage that results in degenerative changes in the body's cells. The degree of oxidative stress and cell damage that a body experiences are impacted by diet and lifestyle choices, such as substance use. His research also shows that as we age, the NAD+ levels in our bodies begin to drop. When that happens certain genetic functions change—functions that are associated with maintaining cell health. Other researchers are investigating the role of NAD+ in DNA repair—an ongoing process given the constant onslaught our bodies are subjected to via stress, environmental toxins, EMFs and RFs, poor diet, and more.[53]

Human trials on NAD+ are under way around the world. These clinical trials are being led by Dr. Grant in Sydney, my husband and clinical director, Dr. Richard Mestayer at Springfield Wellness Center, and scientists at The New Orleans Bio Innovation Center through NAD+ Research, Inc., and scientists at many other institutions. For example, pilot studies show that intravenous BR+NAD™ treatment reduces biomarkers

---

[53] Hassina Massudi, Ross Grant, Nady Braidy, Jade Guest, Bruce Farnsworth, Gilles J. Guillemin. Age-Associated Changes In Oxidative Stress and NAD+ Metabolism In Human Tissue. Published: July 27, 2012 http://dx.doi.org/10.1371/journal.pone.0042357

reflective of inflammation in both alcohol and opiate detox patients, while increasing NAD+ levels and improving NAD+/NADH ratio in plasma, which increases NAD+ effectiveness.

Another study under way at NAD+ Research Inc., in collaboration with the Australasian Research Institute, is investigating the pharmacokinetic dynamics of intravenous NAD+ in healthy individuals. Establishing what NAD+ levels are in healthy males age 35-55 will enable us to determine when NAD+ levels are deficient in others.

Also, our trained clinical Fellows continue to document their work treating addicts and alcoholics with safe, rapid, and effective detoxification through BR+NAD™.

Could NAD+ deficiency be the *cause* of addiction?

At Springfield Wellness Center, we understand that addiction depletes the body's store of NAD+ and that NAD+ deficiency is thus a consequence of addiction. However, there are some researchers—including the late Dr. Hoffer, Dr. Theo Verwey, and others who believe that—for some people at least—NAD+ energy deficiency—or NED—is a physical *cause* of addiction.

Physicians are also employing NAD+ in their research and treatment into a variety of other health conditions—ranging from obesity and diabetes to chronic fatigue and Parkinson's. Dr. David Sinclair, for example, who is co-director of the Paul F. Glenn Laboratories for the Biological Mechanisms of Aging at Harvard Medical School, in 2002 discovered a key role of NAD+ biosynthesis in aging.[54] By raising NAD+ levels in his

---

[54] Michael S. Bonkowsi, David A. Sinclair. Slowing aging by design: the rise of NAD' and sirtuin-activating compounds. Nature Reviews Molecular Cell Biology

laboratory animals, his lab was able to slow the aging process over his control group.

So, it appears that NAD+ deficiency may be implicated in a wide range of degenerative diseases—from Alzheimer's and Parkinson's to chronic fatigue, fibromyalgia, and even aging itself. Without adequate NAD+ and mitochondrial function, patients experience fatigue, depression, anxiety, psychosis, neuronal degeneration, memory problems, and increased susceptibility to genetic and epigenetic mutations and disease. Although much more research is needed to understand just how NAD+ impacts these conditions, one thing is certain: all of us working with BR+NAD™ are taking it as a nutritional supplement via nasal spray, transdermal patch, NAD+ cream, or subcutaneous shot! While not as effective as BR+NAD™ administered intravenously, these delivery mechanisms bypass the destructive effects of digestion so that BR+NAD™ is available where it is needed: at the cellular level.

In addition to the personal case studies I've shared with you here—and hundreds more—our study presented to the Society of Neuroscience in 2014 by researchers Broom, Carson, Cook, Hotard, Mestayer, Norris, Simone & Stuller described 60 adult patients (male and female) with addictions to alcohol or opiates whose cravings fell from an average of 5 or 6 (on a 0 to 10 scale) on Day 1 to a rating of two by Day 5, and to one or less by Day 10. Treatment consisted of intravenous infusions of BR+NAD™, supplemented orally with vitamins, amino acids, and N-acetyl cysteine (NAC) for an average of 10 consecutive days. The treatment was administered from 5 to 10 hours daily at individually prescribed dosages of NAD+ each day. Perhaps even more impressive than the initial reduction in cravings, cravings remained low (a rating of 2 or less) 20 months post-treatment.

17, 679–690 (2016) doi:10.1038/nrm.2016.93

*The greater danger for most of us lies not in setting
our aim too high and falling short; but in setting
our aim too low, and achieving our mark.*
—Michelangelo

Current research we are conducting into NAD+

To help us better understand how NAD+ is able to help the body recover from alcohol and drug addiction, we have created our own independent research laboratory, NAD+ Research, Inc., which is housed in New Orleans' Bio Innovation Center. There, we are conducting research into the effects of alcohol consumption on NAD+ and inflammation levels, the effect of intravenous NAD+ on reducing inflammation levels in addiction patients, and the ability of intravenous NAD+ infusions to improve the efficiency of NAD+ transport through the body. The following graphs illustrate the results of our research to date (spring 2018).

CRAVINGS STUDY
By Springfield Wellness Center

Introduction

Treatment of substance abuse disorders continues to challenge clinicians and "cravings" for the abused substance are often impediments to sobriety. Nicotinamide Adenine Dinucleotide (NAD+) has been used in the past with claims of having anti-craving properties. Previous data from this clinic using a similar formulation of NAD+ support the use of NAD+ as a valid treatment for drug cravings. This pilot study retrospectively examined the anti-craving properties of NAD+ in a group of 60 patients. Additionally, patients were assessed on severity of cravings and relapse episodes at 12-20 months post treatment.

Method

The patients were adult males and females with addictions to primarily opiates or alcohol (N=60). Six patients were omitted due to incomplete data. The treatment, Brain Restoration Plus (BR+)™ comprised of IV infusions of NAD+ as well as vitamins, oral amino acids, NAC and variable PRN medications for an average of 10 consecutive days ranging from 5 to 10 hours daily at a dose range of 500mg-1500mg each day. Self-reported craving ratings (0-10 Scale) were collected on Day 1 (before starting treatment), Day 5, and on Day 10 (last day of treatment). Follow up phone surveys were conducted from 12-20 months post treatment (N= 27). Patients reported severity of cravings (1-5) and number of relapse episodes at the present time.

Conclusion

1) NAD+ is an effective detox treatment for alcohol and opiate addicts as evidenced by a significant reduction in craving ratings.
2) NAD+ was effective in reducing and maintaining the number of relapse episodes, as well as severity of drug cravings.
3) NAD+ shows potential as a long-term therapy in maintaining sobriety through minimizing drug cravings and preventing relapse.

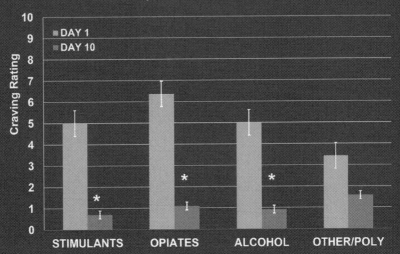

Figure 1. NTR™ Significantly Reduced Craving Ratings for Stimulants, Opiates and Alcohol Groups.

Data from Previous Experiment (2008). Pairwise T-tests Conducted on Stimulant s (n=10), Opiates (n=11), Alcohol (n=12), and Other/Poly (n=7) Groups Following 10 Days of NTR™ Treatment. * indicates p < 0.01.

Figure 2. NAD Significantly Reduces Craving Ratings Associated With Opiate and Alcohol Withdrawal At Five And Ten Days of Treatment

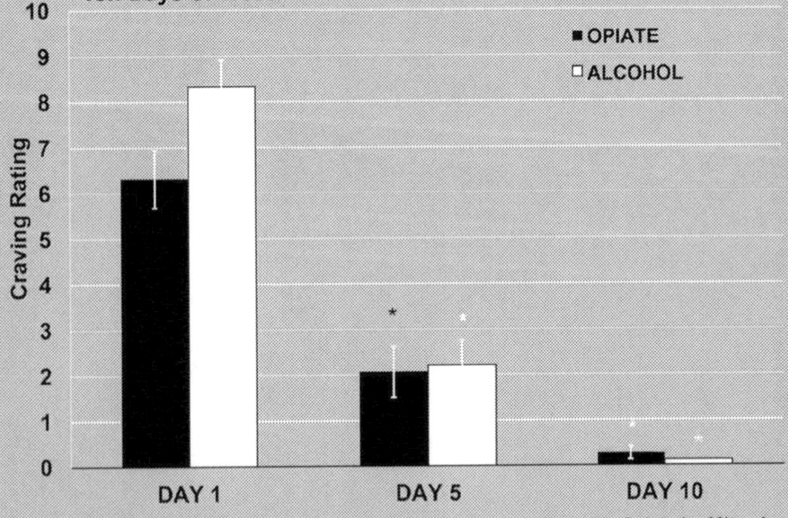

Pairwise T- tests Conducted on Day 1 vs Day 5 and Day 1 vs Day 10 in Opiate (n=29) and Alcohol (n=24) Groups. * indicates p < 0.01.

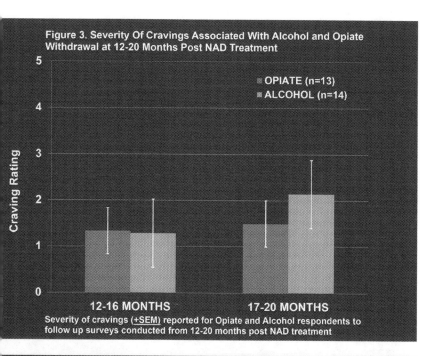

Figure 3. Severity Of Cravings Associated With Alcohol and Opiate Withdrawal at 12-20 Months Post NAD Treatment

Severity of cravings (+SEM) reported for Opiate and Alcohol respondents to follow up surveys conducted from 12-20 months post NAD treatment

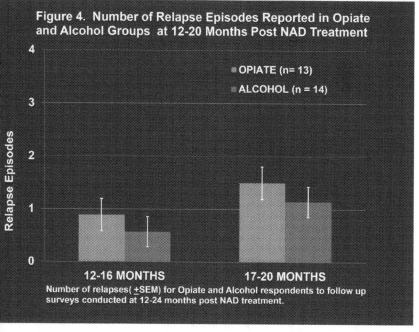

Figure 4. Number of Relapse Episodes Reported in Opiate and Alcohol Groups at 12-20 Months Post NAD Treatment

Number of relapses(+SEM) for Opiate and Alcohol respondents to follow up surveys conducted at 12-24 months post NAD treatment.

Acknowledgements: Thank you to Springfield Wellness Center for providing patient data. Thank you to William Carey University for providing a Professional Development Grant in support of this project.

Brief Substance Craving Scale Results with Alcohol Addicted Patients

The following results were achieved by obtaining subjective data form the patients treated at Springfield Wellness Center for alcohol addiction using BR+. Patients were asked to complete a scale, rating the intensity, frequency and length of their Cravings (consuming desire to use). Ratings were then scored on a scale of 0 to 12 (0 meaning no cravings; 12 meaning the patient was experiencing severe cravings).

Pt. ID #	Day 1	Day 5	Last Day of Tx	Notes
141	12	0	0	8 days of treatment
153	8	4	0	8 days of treatment
149	4	3	0	10 days of treatment
151	10	3	0	7 days of treatment
154	5	0	0	8 days of treatment
145	10	7	3	11 days of treatment
163	6	3	0	9 days of treatment
165	8	0	0	10 days of treatment
176	8	3	0	10 days of treatment
177	12	0	0	10 days of treatment
183	6	4	0	10 days of treatment
190	12	0	0	10 days of treatment

Brief Substance Craving Scale Results with Opiate Addicted Patients

The following results were achieved by obtaining subjective data form the patients treated at Springfield Wellness Center for opiate addiction using BR+. Patients were asked to complete a scale, rating the intensity, frequency and length of their Cravings (consuming desire to use). Ratings were then scored on a scale of 0 to 12 (0 meaning no cravings; 12 meaning the patient was experiencing severe cravings).

Pt. ID #	Day 1	Day 5	Last Day of Tx	Notes
143	8	4	1	8 days of treatment
159	7	0	0	10 days of treatment
161	6	1	0	9 days of treatment
162	11	0	0	7 days of treatment
169	10	0	0	10 days of treatment
174	7	0	0	10 days of treatment
175	3	0	0	10 days of treatment
182	12	0	0	10 days of treatment
184	8	3	0	10 days of treatment
150	5	4	3	8 days of treatment

BR+NAD™ REDUCES OXIDATIVE STRESS
By Springfield Wellness Center

This is pilot data from the lab at Springfield Wellness Center sponsored by NAD Research Inc.

We are still gathering data to get to publishable findings.

A chart shows a dramatic reduction in 8 isoprostane with IV NAD this is a well-established marker for oxidative stress,

B charts show improvements in NAD+ levels and NAD+/NADH ratio all graphs demonstrate the antioxidant power of IV NAD+.

Response to intravenous NAD+ Therapy in Subjects Treated for:

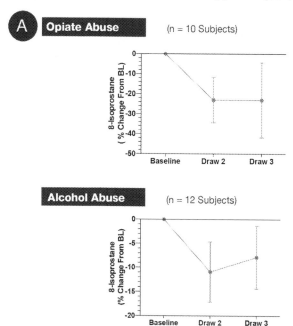

B **Response to intravenous NAD+ Therapy in Subjects Treated for:**

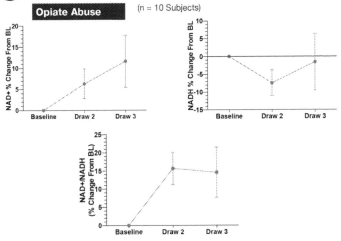

Opiate Abuse (n = 10 Subjects)

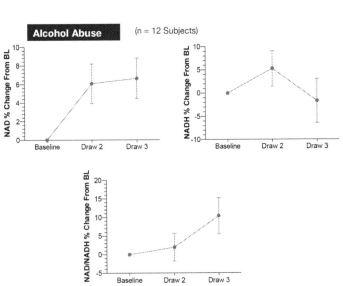

Alcohol Abuse (n = 12 Subjects)

The following pages are selected graphs
from Dr. Mestayer's presentation at
the 2017 LASCAT Conference.

What is NAD+ used for?

This diagram shows what we know of the many functions that NAD+ performs in healthy cells. NAD+ is essential in cell energy production—without which cells cannot do their work. It is involved in DNA repair and gene expression—the process by which genes are turned on and off. It is included in cell signaling, immune function, and the production of vital enzymes. It probably is involved in increasing the length of telomeres, which has anti-aging benefits. NAD+ is also thought to be a neurotransmitter. Any one of these functions would be necessary, but the fact that NAD+ is involved in so many of them highlights the significance of this molecule and shows that prolonged depleted NAD+ levels can have profound health consequences. Just how the body prioritizes which NAD+ functions it will carry out if levels are insufficient for all of them is another fertile area for research.

What is NAD+ Used for?

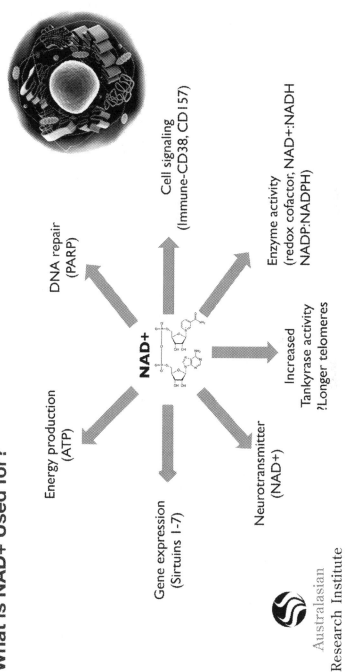

* *Pilot studies continue to explore these markers with the hope of generating clinical trials.*

Australasian
Research Institute

Energy production (ATP)

Gene expression (Sirtuins 1-7)

DNA repair (PARP)

Cell signaling (Immune-CD38, CD157)

NAD+

Neurotransmitter (NAD+)

Increased Tankyrase activity ?Longer telomeres

Enzyme activity (redox cofactor; NAD+:NADH NADP:NADPH)

163

Alcohol's effect on NAD+ levels and inflammation

This diagram shows alcohol consumption greater than one drink/day decreases levels of NAD+ in the brain and increases inflammation as measured by readings of cerebrospinal fluid. With an intake greater than one alcoholic drink/day, average cerebrospinal NAD+ levels begin to drop, while cerebrospinal fluid levels of interleukin-6 (IL-6), which is a marker for inflammation, begin to rise. Alcohol's effect on both NAD+ levels and inflammation in the cerebrospinal fluid is likely reflective of NAD+ activity in the brain.

Alcohol ↓ brain NAD⁺ & ↑ inflam.

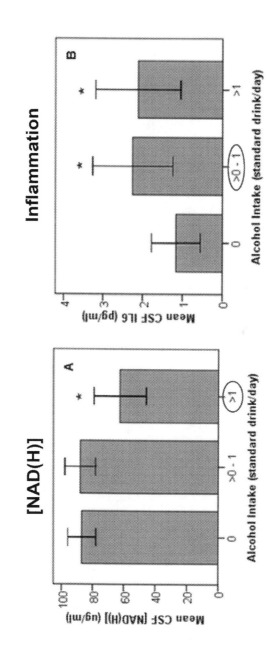

Guest et al PLoS ONE 9(1):e85335. 2014

* *Pilot studies continue to explore these markers with the hope of generating clinical trials.*

Intravenous NAD+ infusion reduces inflammation levels in addiction patients

This diagram shows the results of a pilot study that compared NAD+ plasma levels in 30 healthy participants with NAD+ plasma levels in 26 alcohol patients and 19 opiate patients, matched by age and gender. At the study's outset, levels of 8-isoprostane, a biomarker for oxidative stress, are higher in the addiction patients—both the alcohol and the opiate patients. After four days of intravenous BR+NAD™ therapy, another reading of plasma levels begins showing a dramatic reduction in the oxidative stress marker in both the alcohol patients and the opiate patients. For opiate patients, the levels of 8-isoprostane continue to drop all the way to the last day of treatment, while the decline of the oxidative stress marker in alcohol patients tends to level off after Day 8, 9, or 10. This is a significant finding that warrants further research.

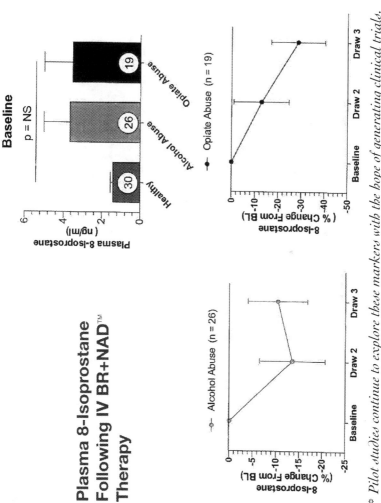

Plasma 8-Isoprostane Following IV BR+NAD™ Therapy

Baseline

p = NS

Plasma 8-isoprostane (ng/ml)

Healthy (30) · Alcohol Abuse (26) · Opiate Abuse (19)

—●— Opiate Abuse (n = 19)

8-Isoprostane (% Change From BL)

Baseline · Draw 2 · Draw 3

—○— Alcohol Abuse (n = 26)

8-Isoprostane (% Change From BL)

Baseline · Draw 2 · Draw 3

Pilot studies continue to explore these markers with the hope of generating clinical trials.

167

Intravenous NAD+ infusion reduces a second inflammation marker in addiction patients

The results from this pilot study show that levels of plasma TNF-alpha, a biomarker for inflammation, are higher in alcohol and opiate patients than in healthy patients, and higher in alcohol patients than opiate patients. It also shows that TNF-alpha levels respond positively following four days of intravenous BR+NAD™ therapy. The graph also indicates that for alcohol patients, the drop in TNF-alpha tends to level off by the third blood draw, which is on day 8, 9, or 10. In the opiate patients, however, we see a continued drop in TNF-alpha on the third blood draw, which is at the end of the BR+NAD™ treatment. It is interesting that, here again, we see two different patterns of reduction, which is also seen in the 8-isoprostane level drops. In both cases, we have shown that intravenous NAD+ helps reduce markers of inflammation.

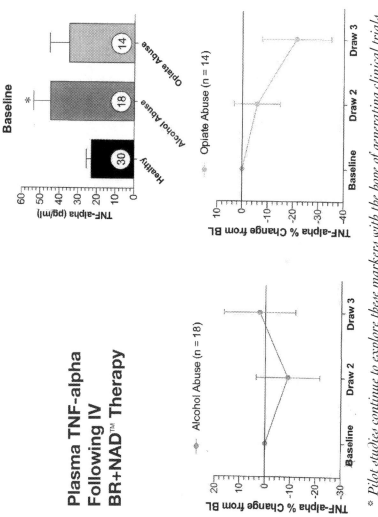

Plasma TNF-alpha Following IV BR+NAD™ Therapy

Baseline

TNF-alpha (pg/ml)

Healthy (30) · Alcohol Abuse (18) * · Opiate Abuse (14)

Alcohol Abuse (n = 18)

TNF-alpha % Change from BL

Baseline · Draw 2 · Draw 3

Opiate Abuse (n = 14)

TNF-alpha % Change from BL

Baseline · Draw 2 · Draw 3

Pilot studies continue to explore these markers with the hope of generating clinical trials.

Intravenous BR+NAD™ infusions increase NAD+/NADH ratio in alcohol abuse patients

Again, this diagram shows pilot data of the response to intravenous BR+NAD™ in 19 subjects treated for alcohol abuse. What is significant in this diagram, in addition to the rise in NAD+ plasma levels after four days of treatment, a higher NAD+/NADH ratio, suggests a better utilization of NAD+ will occur. This warrants additional research to be followed up in clinical trials.

Response to Intravenous BR+NAD™ Therapy in Subjects Treated for Alcohol Abuse

(n = 19 Subjects)

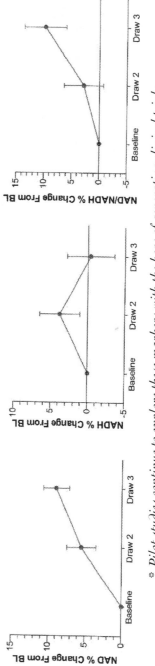

* *Pilot studies continue to explore these markers with the hope of generating clinical trials.*

Intravenous BR+NAD™ infusions increase NAD+/NADH ratio in opiate addiction patients

As in the previous diagram, this one shows pilot data of the response to intravenous BR+NAD™ for 17 subjects treated for opiate addiction. After four days of intravenous BR+NAD™ treatment, NAD+ levels have risen in plasma; NADH levels have dropped; and the ratio of NAD+/NADH has increased, which we believe is significant. Again, this is unpublished pilot data, which could be used to design a more comprehensive study.

Response to Intravenous BR+NAD™ Therapy in Subjects Treated for Opiate Abuse

(n = 17 Subjects)

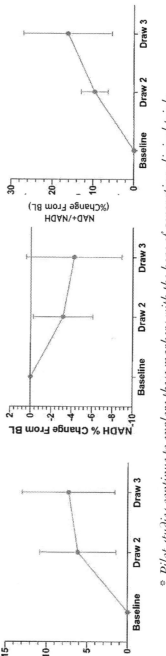

Pilot studies continue to explore these markers with the hope of generating clinical trials.

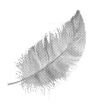

Continuous effort—not strength or intelligence—
is the key to unlocking our potentials.
—Winston Churchill

CHAPTER THIRTEEN

Resources for Spreading the Health

In order to make the benefits of intravenous BR+NAD™ available to as many patients as possible, we have offered a training program for other healthcare professionals since 2013. Physicians, therapists, and nurses who complete the training become certified Fellows of BR+MD Consultants™. They complete an intense, two-day on-site apprenticeship to become versed in our patient intake, prescription formulation, and administration protocols and the standards of practice we have developed over our many years of clinical observations and continuing research. The remainder of the 12-month program takes place at trainees' locations, under the close supervision of our faculty, who are committed to helping clinicians excel in improving their patients' lives through this treatment option.

A key component of Fellow certification is the pledge to administer BR+NAD™ compounded by Archway Apothecary exclusively. This is the only way of ensuring that patients receive the 99% pure NAD+ upon which our treatment protocols and outcomes are based.

Fellows further affirm their commitment to providing

compassionate care of the highest standard to individuals and families experiencing the emotional and/or physical consequences of addiction, substance abuse, anxiety, bereavement, depression, acute, chronic or post-traumatic stress, chronic pain, and neurodegenerative diseases associated with aging. Because the brain mediates everything—body, mind, and spirit—by restoring brain health we positively impact those seeking physical, emotional, and spiritual well-being. Respectful listening to a patient's story can begin the healing process through the establishment of trust. Authentic compassion is paramount and, along with truth and integrity, is the hallmark of treatment success. Our motto is, "No guilt, no shame, and no judgment."

In addition to responsibly sharing this life-changing treatment option, we believe it is good for patient care and the advancement of medical knowledge to build collaborative relationships with those who study with us. We chose the name "Fellows" intentionally, because our relationships with Fellows do not end upon completion of the training program. Rather, they become part of our network of professionals sharing clinical updates and research advances so that, together, we remain good stewards of this breakthrough treatment option.

If you are a healthcare provider who would like to become a BR+NAD™ Fellow, please contact us by calling 1-225-294-5955. or visit www.brplusnad.com.

For those who require privacy

While we believe there should be no more shame associated with seeking treatment for addiction than seeking it for any other illness, there are some individuals for whom the need to keep treatment confidential is nevertheless paramount. At

Springfield Wellness Center, we strive to accommodate these individuals by designing private treatment sessions. Contact us to find out more about our private Concierge Service.

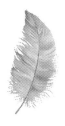

*Forgiveness is not always easy. At times, it feels more painful
than the wound we suffered, to forgive the one that inflicted
it. And yet, there is no peace without forgiveness.*
—Marianne Williamson

CHAPTER FOURTEEN

There Are Angels Among Us

Oh, I believe there are angels among us sent
down to us from someplace up above.

They come to you and me in our darkest hours, to show us how to
live, to teach us how to give, to guide us with the light of love.

—Don Goodman and Becky Hobbs, recorded by Alabama

I discovered in my first dark night of the soul that it isn't easy to recognize the angels among us. Our pain is so self-consuming that we do not recognize the gifts of kindness from strangers until we emerge into the light of redemption. One part of me is reticent to share my experiences of encountering the angels, but another part encourages me to do so in case my stories may provide hope to someone else who feels hopeless in their dark night.

A dear friend who is a devout Catholic had several operations on his neck that ultimately led to an opiate addiction. Before taking our BR+NAD™ treatment, he suffered immense pain. His health continued to decline both physically and mentally with the commensurate loss of hope that can accompany years of suffering. One day he confessed to me that "the only time I have seriously considered suicide was when I was detoxing on my own. I found myself in the darkest place I have ever been with a sense that there was no way out." His description of his own "dark night" was so poignant that I share it with others to help them see that we can, and do, get to the other side. It is very difficult to believe there is hope when there is little or no light. That is why we have angels among us. Our dark nights are the ultimate test of faith and personal triumph. We are meant to persevere in facing the incremental deaths of the ego. As grace would have it, it's when we feel the most alone that we meet the angels who walk among us!

As for my dark night of the soul, during the early years after losing my marriage and my father I wandered around in a daze. I often felt like I was trapped in a bell jar. I could see people talking to me, but I really couldn't hear what they were saying. It was muffled until I could shake myself long enough to give some audible response.

Once I found out about my husband's infidelity, I decided to go to Europe for the summer. I did not tell my husband that I knew he planned to take another woman with him on his search for a Zen master. I only found out the night before I was to leave. My decision to keep this knowledge to myself instead of confronting him may have been a mistake, but it was what I decided to do, believing circumstances had to play themselves out if they had gone this far.

I know that alcohol and drug use played a role in the dissolution of our marriage. I was too young and naïve to understand the impact at the time. Addiction shows no mercy!

Those three months in Europe were filled with tears. I traveled everywhere on a Eurail pass and saw magnificent sights through the lens of depression. My thoughts were tortuous. All I could think was of them being intimate, or wondering what I had done wrong. I prayed all the time. I don't think I passed a chapel, church, cathedral, or basilica without going inside to light a candle with a prayer for my marriage to survive.

It was a sunny morning when I arrived in sultry Venice, where the scent of salty air welcomed me. I got off the train with my backpack and eventually found the hostel where I planned to stay. It was lodging offered through a convent so I knew I would be safe. The nuns were friendly and seemed to realize that I was hiding my sadness. Their compassionate eyes gave them away. They were very helpful with informing me of the policies of curfew, shower use, and meals. After settling into my room, I decided I would walk to Piazza San Marco.

Making my way through the narrow streets of Venice was sensual in the warm afternoon breeze. The old stones, salty air, and blue sky caught my tearful attention. I wiped my eyes as I entered the Piazza. It was overwhelming. It was beautiful. It was BIG. It was also OLD. The history in this one place was more than I had ever experienced. I was in awe. I was also lonely.

As I made my way among the people, I found a small venue selling wine and cheese under the portico facing the Piazza. I took a seat at a small round table tucked away in a corner. I ordered a glass of wine and began watching the people, hundreds of them, strolling around the square. Of course, I noticed the couples walking hand in hand, arm in arm, smiling, laughing, soaking up the summer's day without worry. No one was rushing. It was peaceful, with beautiful music riding the breeze from the small string ensembles meandering among the tables. I wanted to share this with my husband, but he wasn't there. It was in that moment of emptiness that I noticed the birds—pigeons—lots of them!

Flocks of pigeons would take flight and land as people walked around. I noticed that a member of one flock fell over each time it landed. Once I realized the little bird needed help, I became hyper-focused on this particular flock. I lost awareness of the people walking around and simply kept my eyes on the flock. I got up from the table and walked out onto the Piazza, my eyes trained on this specific group of birds. With each landing, I got closer and closer and was able to identify the wounded bird. Keeping my eye on that bird, I was able to estimate where he might land next. When he did, I was close enough to bend down and grab him before the flock flew away again. He was flapping his wings trying to get away when I discovered why he kept falling over. His legs were bound by wire that is used to prevent the birds from nesting in St. Mark's Basilica.

So here I was in the middle of the Piazza with a wild pigeon in my hands when I looked up and realized a small crowd was forming. I must have heard seven different languages as I stood there asking if anyone had a pair of scissors to cut the wire. One woman took a pair of manicuring scissors from her purse and came over to help me. I held the pigeon as she gently cut the wire, pulling it from his swollen legs and feet. Once the wire was removed, I gently tossed the bird into the air and watched him fly away. The small group of spectators clapped and cheered. I blushed, smiled and thanked the woman who helped and quietly walked back to my table. I do not know that woman's name. Our only connection was the brief time during which we shared this experience. I like to think she was an angel among us. That summer I had several angel encounters as I traveled throughout the European countryside. A young man named Peter was one. A student of Count Von Durkheim, he helped me find my way to the Black Forest when I was lost. Another angel was the young unnamed Italian gentleman on a crowded train from Florence to Brindisi, who saw the tears running down my face and helped me find a safe place to rest during the night, on the sink in the water closet as he guarded the door. Two more were a mother and daughter in Budapest who invited me to have dinner with them so I would not dine alone. Still, another was an unknown gentleman at a formal black-tie ball sitting in front of me with his friends. As I sniffled in the darkness behind him, he gently, without turning around, simply patted the side of my knee to offer assurance. Each of these strangers graced me with their mercy in my time of need. So, did that little bird. His message to me was that you can fly even through you are bound. You don't give up. You try again and again until what binds you is cut. Once unbound you are free to fly as you were meant to fly....on the wings of wisdom and Grace. Have faith. Be tenacious, be audacious, even be bodacious in your dark night and you will find your way to the light.

That is my message to each person I meet in our clinic: Don't ever give up or give into despair! Every person who suffers from addiction and every family member who suffers with them needs to know there is hope. It doesn't matter how many residential programs, intensive outpatient programs, partial hospital programs, individual counseling sessions, 12-step programs, AA meetings, or any combination of them all, you have tried. Very little changes until the well-meaning professionals, family members and YOU understand that addiction is first a brain disease. That which can free you is BR+NAD™, but you must have faith that you *will* fly, unbound, once your cravings and withdrawals have been defeated.

Life has a way of teaching us the lessons we need to learn to grow. It is easy to feel good and strong when things are going our way. But we grow by facing the challenges life presents when things are not going our way. We must develop discipline, a practice, in strengthening the physical, psychological, and spiritual parts of ourselves that enable us to overcome these challenges. BR+NAD™ can help, restoring the brain and giving us the clarity and confidence to do what we need to do.

So many who suffer the modern-day scourge of addiction know all too well what being consumed by fear will do. When cravings or withdrawals begin, and you know only one way to get relief—the drug—you will find a way to get it, no matter what. The misconception that an addict is always "looking for the high" no longer applies once the true grip of addiction has invaded body, mind, and soul. Addicts are looking for relief—even though the relief is only temporary and the price is very high. It is not only the price per dose that is exacted, but the price in self-esteem, guilt, shame, confusion, lost relationships, jobs, and health. The price can be so high that some fear they will never be able to recover; but I have seen again and again that they can and do, once they face their fears.

Most of us have a very difficult time admitting we even have fears, much less face them, but doing so is an *absolute prerequisite* to freedom. Only then will you discover that you are stronger and more courageous than you ever thought possible. With this new awareness of your strength and courage, you can manage your health while you travel the road to your destiny.

Most of the people who come to us for treatment are skeptics. They have tried every option available and with their last exhausted breath take the chance that what we claim may be true. They are desperate, hopeless, and afraid, but they show up anyway. Little do they know that the commitment they make for the 10 short days of our BR+NAD™ detox treatment will mark the beginning of their new life. It is not a cure. It requires a commitment to wellness management and maintenance. It requires lifestyle changes that must become the "new normal," with the acknowledgment that "stress management" is essential for mid-brain health. In India, Ayurveda medicine teaches the importance of prevention. It is healthy to bathe your senses with beauty: look at beautiful things, listen to beautiful things, touch beautiful things, taste beautiful things, smell beautiful things. It is also healthy to keep good company!

Rogers and Hammerstein wrote a song in 1945 for the Broadway musical, *Carousel*. At that time, my father had returned home after fighting in WWII. The war was over, and the enemy was defeated. I was born a year later which makes me a "baby boomer." For those of you too young to know why we were given that name I'll save you the trouble of asking your "device" for the answer. There were thousands of babies being born after the war because our brave military men and women came home by the thousands to the loving arms of their spouses or sweethearts. Birthrates skyrocketed. Alcohol consumption skyrocketed, as well. The scars of war were difficult to manage, but families stayed together in tough times back then, even when the remedy in a bottle of whiskey caused another kind of pain. When I was a child, I remember asking my father if I could have a sip of what he was drinking. He said it was his *medicine* and politely said no.

A significant number of us became "adult children of alcoholics," but we would not admit our family secret for years. Alcoholics Anonymous was the only venue for help at that time, and proud military officers would die before admitting they needed help. And, that is what happened. My father died before admitting he needed help. That is why I have written this book: to inform and to encourage. I don't want anyone else to die rather than admitting they need help. Fight for your life! Let go of the guilt and shame that binds you. Even if you are bound, you can fly. Just keep trying until your prayers are answered and what binds you is cut! And remember this: You are not your disease. You *have* a disease. Diseases can be cured or managed. Do not define yourself as a disease!

Lastly, and most importantly, this is what I want you to remember. There is an angel I know about on Mt. Whitney in California who silently sings these words to all of us in our time of need.

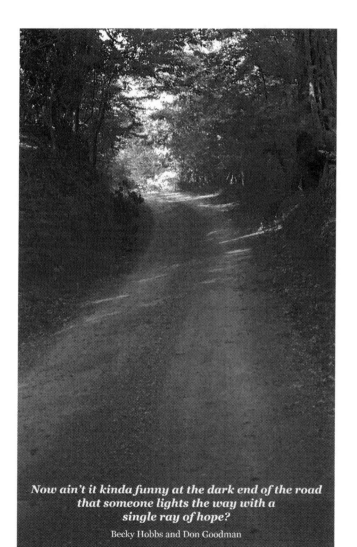

Now ain't it kinda funny at the dark end of the road
that someone lights the way with a
single ray of hope?

Becky Hobbs and Don Goodman

Paula Norris Mestayer, M.Ed., LPC, FAPA

Paula Norris Mestayer was an educator for 11 years after graduating from LSU in 1969. She completed graduate degrees in education and independent study in psychotherapy from Tulane University before taking her clinical internship at the Manhattan Children's Psychiatric Hospital. She has devoted her professional life to helping patients deal effectively with a wide variety of sub-acute psycho-physiological conditions, including panic and anxiety disorders, chronic and acute stress, depression and bereavement, alcohol and substance abuse and marital and family challenges. For 22 years she was a consultant at Ochsner Foundation Hospital with the Behavioral Health and Addiction Treatment Units. Concurrently, 11 of those years she was the director of a private nonprofit residential program for abused and neglected children. In 2001, she founded an outpatient clinic providing services for the treatment of chemical dependency and acute stress utilizing intravenous infusions, which then led to the development of BR+NAD at Springfield Wellness Center.

Paula Norris Mestayer is a Licensed Professional Counselor (LPC), a Fellow of the American Psychotherapy Association (FAPA), and a member of the American Counseling Association and the Louisiana Counseling Association. She was certified by the International Society of Clinical Hypnosis, The New Orleans

Society of Clinical Hypnosis, the PAIRS Foundation for Marital Family Therapy, and the ADTR-Creative Arts Therapy.

She lives with her loving husband, Dr. Richard Mestayer, III, in Natchez, Mississippi with her horses, dogs, chickens, ducks, cat, donkey and their visiting children (5) and grandchildren (8).

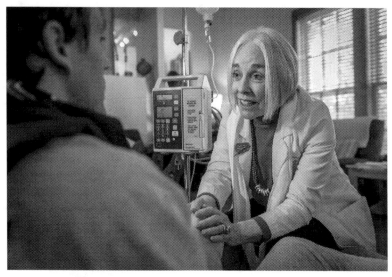

Paula Mestayer encouraging a patient at Springfield Wellness Center.

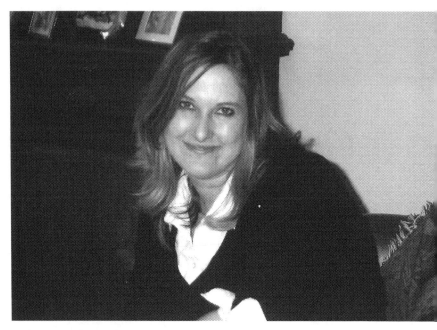

Miranda Norris Baham post-treatment from the William Hitt Cent[e]

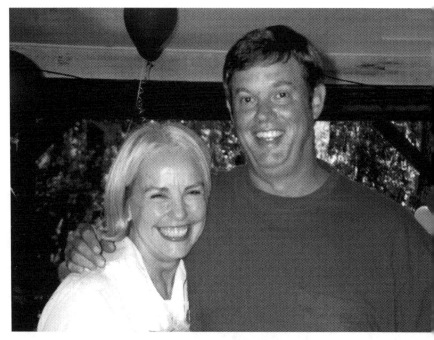

Paula and Richard Mestayer

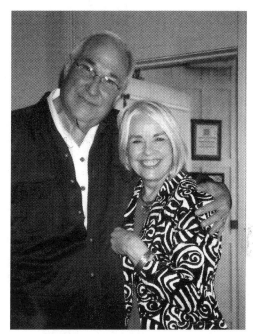

Willam Hitt and Paula Mestayer
at Springfield Wellness Center

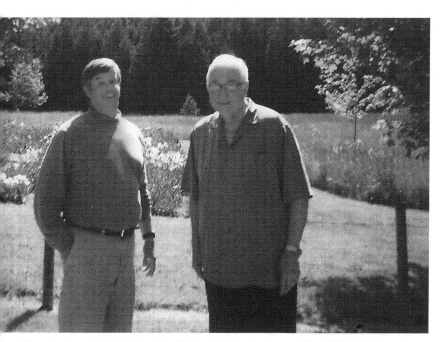

Two Amigos on holiday, Dr. Richard Mestayer and Dr. William Hitt

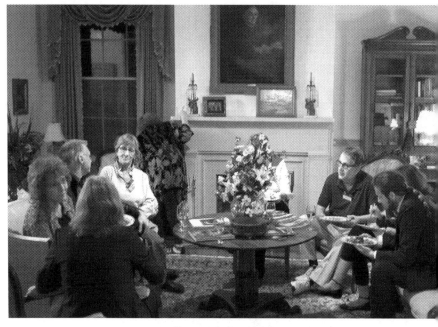

Pre-summit gathering

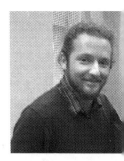

Dr. Nady Braidy, Australaisan Research Institute at the Brain Restoration Summit 20

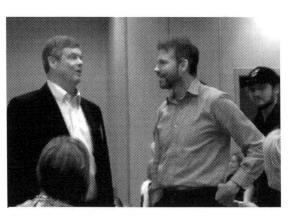

Dr. Mestayer and Dr. Ross Grant, Australaisan Research Institute, at the Brain Restoration Summit 2015

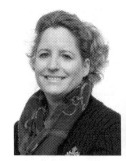

Dr. Elizabeth Stuller first BR+ Fellow and renown psychiatrist

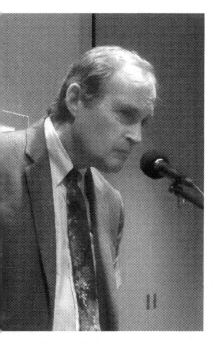

James Watson listens to a question at the 2015 Summit

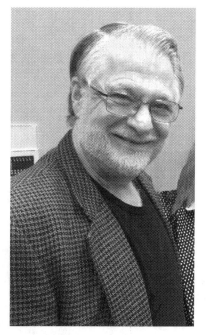

Louis Cataldie, MD, author of *10,000 Addicts Later* and speaker at 2015 Summit

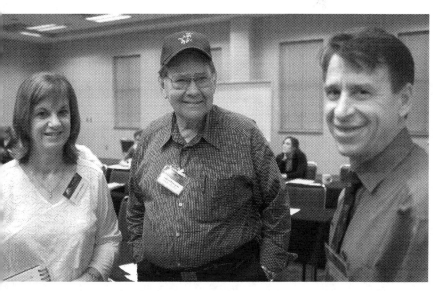

Camille and Addison Thompson with Dr. John Sturges, 2015 Summit

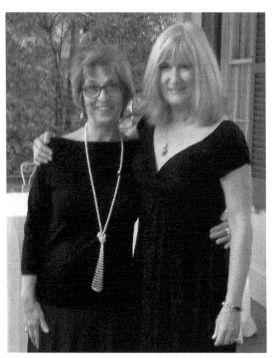

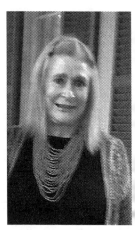

Lourdes Corbala
William Hitt Center

Theresa Norris and Leslee Goodman
at Summit reception

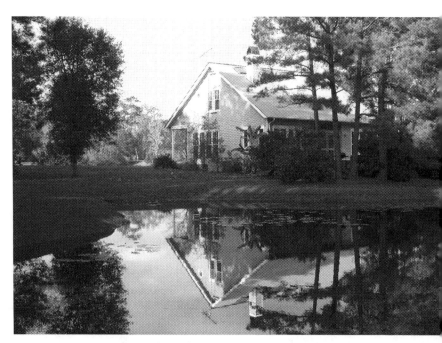

Springfield Wellness Center of Louisiana

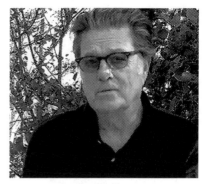

Garland Robinette

July 14, 2018   10:38pm
A text message to Paula Mestayer from Garland Robinette concerning a dear
friend

Paula, how gently you must sleep knowing the souls you've saved.

I've traveled the world in the bubble of a privileged life. I've been
a janitor, news anchor, VP of an oil company, radio talk guy and an
artist. I've dined with presidents, met with kings, and interviewed
the world's most famous. But I've found that in the backwoods of
Springfield, Louisiana lies the reality of the most important thing in
the world, what Joseph Campbell called "the between of what we
are and WHAT WE SHOULD BE!"

You may never realize what a difference you've made--the
connection with a disappearing thing called love, of which there
is so little left. But no matter, the ones you've touched will never
forget. Hold these souls closely so that you always understand
that what you do is rare."

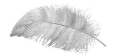

Broken can be beautiful. For it's in that brokenness that we find hope. It's in that hope that we find healing. And it's in that healing that we are made more beautiful and stronger than ever before.
—David Arms

04164332-00961053

Printed in the United States
By Bookmasters